Homeopathy, what to expect?

By Edward De Beukelaer

'When your views on the world and your intellect are being challenged and you begin to feel uncomfortable because of a contradiction you've detected that is threatening your current model of the world or some aspect of it, pay attention. You are about to learn something. This discomfort and intellectual conflict is when learning is taking place.'
William Drury, College of the Atlantic

Trafford rev. 01/03/2019

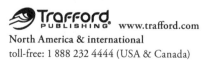 www.trafford.com

North America & international
toll-free: 1 888 232 4444 (USA & Canada)
fax: 812 355 4082

Acknowledgements.

This book is dedicated to all the people that are about to discover homeopathy in the hope that they will make a sensible integration of homeopathy into their medical strategy(ies). I hope it also will bring an interesting message and helpful information to those who are already initiated.

There are many people who made it possible for this book to come to life.

First there is the very active, friendly and encouraging international homeopathic community that makes it possible to learn how to practise homeopathy and that works as a continual stimulus to strive for excellence. A few of its members allowed me to use their case records to make this book more interesting. I am very grateful to them.

It is necessary to make special mention of Dr. Marc Brunson, veterinary surgeon near Liège in Belgium. He is the driving force behind a school called CLH (Centre Liégeois d'Homéopathie) and taught me and many others common sense homeopathy that always aspires to improve without losing sight of the essential homeopathic principles and staying clear of elitism. It is possible that without his input I would never have become a homeopath.

I want to send a special thought to my family, who are so very dear to me and who accepted my many absences during the preparations.

I have to thank Carl Dellaert, my uncle, who suggested the lay-out of the front-page.

Phil Robbins was the dedicated proofreader of the manuscript. His work has been very valuable and much appreciated. There is also a thank you to Rose for important logistic input.

Table of Contents

Introduction

In the last few hundred years modern science has established itself as the gold standard for reliable medicine. Therefore official and peer reviewed information on medicine concerns conventional medicine only. This leaves an open gap for non-conventional medical practitioners sometimes eagerly filled by those who have the best communication skills. The subject of alternative medicine has become as varied as there are different philosophies on healing and cure. Often personal convictions and enthusiasm are ingredients of the available information.

Reading enthusiastic works on different techniques and ideas is a pleasant experience. The enthusiasm of others fuels optimism and belief in solutions. The experiences and opinions of others feed the desire for knowledge and help us in our quest for the ideal medical solution. No medical system is perfect. Different systems will suit different people. Not everybody has the same objective in medicine. The art of medicine is to be reasonable and use the available options in a balanced way to achieve the best results or the results desired. To achieve this it is important to be well informed on the different techniques one wants to choose from.

The purpose of this book is to help in providing sensible guidance. As a vet working with animals, I have the advantage of dealing with unprejudiced patients. This helps to remove some of the hype and placebo effect present in medicine; what you do either works or doesn't work.

Among the various alternative techniques on offer, homeopathic treatment and homeopathic remedies are enjoying a booming interest. The motivations for this interest are diverse. Personal convictions, personal experiences, word of mouth, dissatisfaction with conventional treatments, curiosity, search for more options, demand for less aggressive treatments, search for more efficient treatments, etc., the list of reasons is long.

Whatever the reason, if your eye is drawn to homeopathy or you are already using homeopathic remedies, it is best to have some understanding of this medical technique if you wish to benefit from its potential.

It is easy to get carried away by the spectacular results homeopathic remedies can achieve. It is just as easy to consider homeopathic treatment as totally ineffective when it fails. In the interest of homeopathy and in the interest of patients it is advisable to take an objective look at this prescription technique and the variations on its original concept. This will help to understand the different views on homeopathy and to integrate homeopathic medicine in the best possible way to suit personal choices. Because there is no difference between homeopathy for humans and homeopathy for animals, what follows is applicable to all.

The first part of this book will treat homeopathy from an historical point of view culminating in an effort to explain what constitutes its possibilities and weaknesses and how you can differentiate homeopathy from other non-conventional techniques.

The second part is a compilation of 101 veterinary case records that have been published by thirteen different veterinary homeopaths who have been educated in four different homeopathy schools in Belgium and France. The purpose is to illustrate the power of classical homeopathy and the workings of its daily practice. The cases are selected to illustrate what you can and should expect from homeopathy. Although they are veterinary cases, they have a value as examples for what can be expected from homeopathy for humans.

Obviously all these cases are successful cases. Publishing unsuccessful cases has no real value because we cannot learn from them. All homeopaths have cases for which they haven't found a solution. Unsuccessful cases remind practitioners that their task of increasing their prescription efficiency is ongoing. The successful cases are a living proof that it is worth while pursuing the homeopathic effort for the benefit of the patient and those around him. Some of the cases illustrate brilliant prescriptions, in other cases clients have been very patient.

How I came to homeopathy.

When I graduated as a veterinary surgeon I felt ready to take on any patient that would be presented to me. Teaching in veterinary and medical schools is well structured and offers a rational vision on health and disease. It not only offers a logical vision but because of the scientific and statistic foundation of this knowledge, graduates are also given the impression of possessing the truth on medicine. Anything that deviates from this truth is readily considered as unreliable or imaginary. As a new graduate, I had heard about homeopathy. Because of the confidence given by my education I considered it to be an obscure occupation, a sign of a practitioner straying from the right path.

Like many of my young colleagues the first years in practice consisted of building up experience and finding where to settle. Experience means that, as young graduates, we have to fill the gap between medical education and daily practice. What is taught in medical school is not always readily adaptable to the real world. This is reflected in the discussion between veterinary schools and professional organisations: schools are accused of not preparing students enough for daily practice. Universities argue that their task is to form scientists not practitioners.

University teaches how to learn and develops the knowledge and capacity we can use to adapt to the requirements of patients and clients. Flexibility and openness we have to create for ourselves.

After a few years in practice, a new problem emerged for me: the reality of chronic and recurring disease. Animals would come in time and time again for the same problem. I started to feel inadequate by delivering the same treatments every time they were brought to the surgery. I also started to sense a discrepancy between the diagnostic possibilities that existed and the treatments that were available to me. The proposed treatments for a large variety of diagnoses and symptoms came down to using antibiotics, steroids, non-steroidal anti-inflammation drugs or a combination of them: treatments were often very similar even if the diagnosis was different.

I started to wonder whether there could not be something else to propose to my clients. It did not appear to me that I was finding either satisfying or satisfactory solutions for their animal's problems. I was merely stopping symptoms without curing my patients and I had become a merchant of medicines very much conditioned by the drug companies.

Coincidences often bring things together at the right moment. In the same period of rising dissatisfaction, I received publicity for a book on homeopathy and bought it. I wouldn't recommend this particular book to anybody nowadays but it certainly promised me that there was something out there that I could learn to use to improve my service to patients.

I recalled that my grandfather, a psychiatrist and professor in criminology at the Faculty of Law in Leuven (Belgium), who was also very dedicated to the improvement of psychiatric care for young people, had shown a keen interest in this medical principle towards the end of a very successful professional career and life. He was a highly respected man of great authority in his field; he would not have been interested in homeopathy without good reasons.

Much later after reading some of his work, I understood why homeopathy had appealed to him; he had put much effort in bringing together people who were specialised in different disciplines of the study of man (anthropology) to improve approaches towards psychiatry for the young. This was his pursuit to bring a more holistic approach in the conventional treatment of 'the soul'. Homeopathy fitted in with this idea because of its holistic approach to the use of medicines.

My attention was caught and when an invitation for a homeopathy course arrived in my letterbox, I wanted to find out more and enrolled.

The course was run by a group of practising homeopathic vets. A new world opened up to me. I was taught the homeopathic principles and they were really appealing. The teachers were enthusiastic and I became convinced this was a path to pursue. Although they convinced me of the validity of the homeopathic technique, the differences in opinions and the quarrels between them left me somewhat stranded. After four years (I must have been very motivated!) I was incapable of producing any real results using homeopathic remedies and worse, I didn't really understood what exactly I was doing.

The mist started to clear when I went to a different homeopathy school where classical homeopathy was taught. There, I was provided with the building stones for an appropriate understanding of homeopathy: it became clear how homeopathic remedies interfered in the evolution of health and disease and what the conditions are for obtaining good results using homeopathic remedies. Teaching in the first school aimed at giving easy clues for prescribing homeopathic remedies, the second school aimed at teaching us a good homeopathic remedy selection technique.

When I presented homeopathy to a group of practitioners at the Veterinary University in Ghent (Belgium), I became conscious that there was a need for information on how homeopathy can be part of a sensible attitude that uses the best of both conventional and non-conventional medicine.

By studying many books on homeopathic medicine and from my own experience amassed in two very different homeopathy schools, I discovered that homeopathic medicines are used in various ways.

From the beginning of homeopathy, there have been practitioners who searched for alternative ways to use homeopathically diluted remedies. They were motivated by a desire to find easier or more appealing ways to use homeopathically prepared medicines. The study and application of the homeopathic principles demands much effort and rigour. Others adapted the use of homeopathic remedies to their personal philosophies on medicine.

There is a general confusion between the practice of homeopathy and the use of homeopathically prepared medicines. Prescribing homeopathically prepared remedies does not imply that one observes the homeopathic prescription technique. Homeopathic remedies can be used outside homeopathic prescription.

One really important truth is that the more remedies are selected according to the original homeopathic principles, the more they are appropriate for the patient, the more they are capable of making profoundly efficient changes in the patient. The term classical homeopathy refers to the effort of applying these original homeopathic principles as truthfully as possible. It also refers to efforts made by practitioners to help patients as efficiently as possible for as long a time as possible: to find real and lasting cures for them.

Practising classical homeopathy today, when conventional medicine/science is the 'golden' standard, is difficult because homeopathy doesn't fit very well into what is considered as the correct way of practising medicine. Homeopathy cannot be part of a strategy in conventional medicine; it has to be practised alongside it.

Homeopathy is not a mysterious occupation. It has a clear fundamental principle and a scientific, although original, way of finding the indications for medicines and other substances. Homeopathy has something mysterious about it because of the incomprehensible (by conventional standards) cures it can achieve and because it uses medicines where the materiality of the original substance has often disappeared through the homeopathic preparation method. Science is slowly making progress to give homeopathically prepared substances their status as 'real' medicines. As usual, it will be some time before this will be accepted in the mainstream.

There is great confusion between natural medicine, herbal medicine and homeopathy. Interestingly though, these three ways of medical tradition can all make use of homeopathically prepared remedies but only when the homeopathic principles are applied properly can we consider these medicines to become homeopathic. It is also only in this case that remedies obtain the most spectacular cures.

I will make no distinction between human and veterinary homeopathy. The principles are the same. The attitude towards medicine may be different when working with humans or animals, homeopaths may use symptoms in a different way according to the species but the prescription rules and the remedies are the same and the exigency is the same when successful prescription is the objective. The difference has more to do with medical experience and the affinity one has with regards to one species or another.

Veterinary homeopaths can often learn from human homeopaths and vice versa.

Homeopathy in the light of medical history.

Recordings concerning medicine exist since the beginning of writing. Medical techniques are part of cultural traditions and evolution. When these cultural traditions have been continuous for centuries, medical philosophies that were associated with them had the time to evolve into very elaborate and valuable techniques. Examples are Chinese medicine, acupuncture and Ayurvedic medicine.

The western world has known a more turbulent history. European history reflects influences from ancestry, Greek and Arabic traditions. The change to modern times started in the Renaissance when individual thinking gained importance over science 'controlled' by religion, power and popular traditions. Medicine was one of the sciences practised and treated by the many illustrious thinkers throughout European history. At first, medicine was more a theoretical occupation interested in classifications, explanations and experiments. Just like the other scientific occupations, medicine was part of a cultural evolution enjoyed by the enlightened part of the society. For a long time, the patient did not play a very important role in this evolution.

The beginning of the breakthrough to modern medicine started in the 18th century when one Italian scientist suggested that the science of autopsy should be used to discover what changes disease caused in the body. This would improve understanding of disease and become a base for the development of efficient treatments. Before that, autopsies used to be an academic or exhibition-like occupation, destined to satisfy curiosity and sometimes the standing of the scientists.

Up to the beginning of the 19th century, medical treatments were based on habits, word of mouth, traditions and personal beliefs. Very few treatments were the result of the scientific revolution that had been taking place. The idea of linking 'research' to improve the knowledge on disease as a way to develop new treatments had not been expressed so clearly before.

The 18th, 19th and 20th century produced important technical progress that was applied to improve knowledge of the body. Because the newly emerged form of medical science/thinking assumed that once one can explain and understand disease, rational cures and eradication of

7

disease will be found, all the medical attention in the western world became, and still is, directed to research that should improve our knowledge and therefore efficiency. Our medical heritage is 'controlled' by this relatively new concept, which is the result of rationalism and modern science.

This new medical concept was very theoretical and did not produce any results in the beginning; old traditions continued to offer help to the patients and continuous attempts were made, outside the official bodies, to find efficient therapies. Patients were not interested in theories and explanations; they wanted help. Over the years many alternative techniques developed attempting to fill the void left by official medical practitioners who were directing their principal effort more towards improving knowledge about medicine than developing new and efficient treatments. This is less the case nowadays. Modern medicine has caught up and produced many efficient treatments. But it still has a very theoretical approach and still lives much in the promise of future better treatments. As a consequence, a multitude of different forms of non-conventional medicine still flourish on the High Street and the Internet (i.e. modern High Street).

Homeopathy is one of these alternative techniques developed in an attempt to improve the service to the patient. Homeopathy is born in the same scientific, historic and geographic (Europe) context as conventional medicine. Its principles have been 'discovered' by Hahnemann in the same period that marks the birth of modern medicine.

Another historical fact is that the tradition of homeopathy has been kept alive mostly by practitioners who at first were educated by the official and scientific medical establishment. Although there are now many non-medical homeopathic practitioners, most practitioners are also holders of an official medical degree.

Homeopathy is not some oriental curiosity; it is a product of Western European medical history kept alive by those who have been educated in the modern scientific universities. Since its beginning it has been 'persecuted' by the official medical body. Only very few works on the history of medicine mention the existence of homeopathy and when mentioned, are rarely taken seriously and examined thoroughly.

Homeopathy is also one of the best survivors of all the alternative techniques that have sprung to life over the last 250 years in Europe.

To explain part of both the historical and present difficulties of homeopathic medicine, it is helpful to take a look into the name that is used to refer to modern or scientific medicine: it is called conventional medicine, medicine by convention. Convention means 'by common agreement' or 'accepted custom' (Oxford Dictionary). This indicates that scientific medicine is the form of medicine that is preferred. Preferred has to do with opinion, tradition, more desired. Efficacy and objective value play a lesser role in the establishment of tradition or preference. Vision and opinion on matters, personal sensibilities and a sense of 'security' play a bigger role in the establishment and maintenance of conventions.

As a consequence homeopathy tends to develop itself where there are people who accept the possibility of different views, where there are people prepared to accept that 'convention' is not the only way of doing things. This requires some courage. Stepping away from conventions puts you in a vulnerable position which is something not everybody is willing to do.

For these reasons, homeopathy is often considered as a fringe occupation for people who have strayed from the right path.

It will be necessary to lay aside some of the conventional reflexes that govern your perceptions if you want to benefit from homeopathy. One of the major reflexes that stands in the way of efficient homeopathic practice and is also the cause of the impossibility of incorporating homeopathy into scientific medicine, is our desire to classify the patient (i.e. diagnosis), followed by the logical or best known treatment for the condition. You will discover that this desire always leads to a lesser way of using homeopathic medicines. Homeopathy treats the patient, not the disease. This reflex is so deeply built into our western ways that it is, for most students, one of the big hurdles that needs to be overcome before they become classical homeopaths.

I hope you will enjoy your journey into homeopathy!

Homeopathy, a technique on its own.

Homeopathy was formulated by Samuel Hahnemann in the beginning of the 19th century and gave the individual patient the central importance for successful use of medicines. The importance of this individuality principle cannot be stressed enough. It is a common and natural tendency to try and classify ailments and treatments for facilitation and clarity. Successful homeopaths make daily efforts to keep the individuality principle central in their practice.

To understand this better and appreciate the consequences of individuality in medicine, it is interesting to visit the history of the birth of homeopathy.

Hahnemann the instigator of the homeopathic principles.

Samuel Hahnemann was born in Saxony (Germany) in 1755 and died in Paris in 1843.

He was born into a modest artisan family and was destined to become a manual worker at 14 years of age. Because of his capacity and motivation for studying and his keen interest in many sciences, he received financial help and support from several mentors to pursue further education in high school and later university. When he graduated as a medical doctor he had also acquired the use of six foreign languages (Latin, Greek, Arabic, French, English and Italian) and soon added a good knowledge of all aspects of chemistry, metallurgy, mining, agriculture and hygiene.

Very early on in his career, he was the author of many respected publications treating the different aspects of his knowledge and thinking.

He also translated various historical and contemporary works on medicine, chemistry and agriculture.

As a result of his extended knowledge of medicine and his strong striving for perfectionism he became very critical of official contemporary medical practice. During his time, official medical techniques consisted of bleedings, luke-warm baths, enemas, endless diets, use of toxic substances and purges. They were often dangerous, produced many side effects and were most of the time ineffective. There was never any rationale behind these treatments. They were used because everybody used them, based on tradition. Their efficiency was mainly determined by the importance of the physicist.

He abandoned the techniques he was taught and concentrated on offering advice on hygiene to improve his patient's health. He found out that good hygienic advice was much more reliable and effective to increase patient's health.

> Note: One of the occurrences that motivated Hahnemann to turn his back on conventional treatments was the death of Leopold II, a popular and loved monarch of Austria in 1772. When he fell ill, his doctor practised a bleeding followed by a second and a third bleeding. Still not happy with the results, the physicist practised a fourth bleeding which left the well-respected monarch dead. The circumstances of Leopold's death stirred up the medical world and gave rise to much criticism. It was for Hahnemann further proof of the inefficiency of much of the official medical practice. He wrote that many physicists were more motivated by cultivation of their ego than the well-being of patients.

The side effects of various official medical techniques and medicines were often worse than the original complaints they were used for. This was something Hahnemann could not accept and it motivated him to experiment with ways to reduce the side effects of conventional drugs. He tried this by decreasing doses of medicines (he experimented at length with Mercury, a medicine used for syphilis). His desire to reduce side effects from medicines was very significant when he came to formulate the homeopathic principles.

The first big step towards the discovery of the homeopathic principles happened when Hahnemann translated the Treatise of Materia Medica written by Cullen (1712-1790), a Scottish medical scholar. In the chapter about Cinchona Officinalis, the bark of a Peruvian tree used to treat swamp fever, Cullen wrote that the activity of this drug was due to its astringent effect on the stomach.

Hahnemann had used this drug years before when he suffered from a spell of swamp fever and could not agree with Cullen's statement.

He decided to test the effect of Cinchona on himself, now that he was healthy, to see what effect it produced on the body. This idea of using a medical substance on a healthy person to discover its effects had already been advocated and practised by a few other experimenters in the medical field and it is likely that Hahnemann picked up this idea from his extensive knowledge. (Anton von Störk (1731-1803) and Albrecht von Hallen (1707-1777)). This decision was his first step towards the discovery of homeopathy.

Note: It is interesting to observe how Hahnemann, when he became disillusioned with official medicine, turned towards education in hygiene for his patients. In his experience this was often found to be more effective then techniques he was taught and certainly less damaging for patients. Nowadays there is a big increase in effort by conventional medicine to practise preventative medicine by improving people's habits (food, smoking, exercise). Another word for preventative medicine is hygiene.

Does modern medicine subconsciously recognise its incapacity in treating many ailments and the existence of side effects of many of its treatment protocols and therefore increase its attention towards medicine through hygiene?

Hahnemann's experiments.

After ingestion of a few grams of this tree bark preparation, Cinchona officinalis (better known as China) he experienced its poisoning effects. When the poisoning receded he wrote down every symptom that had occurred. What caught his attention immediately was that the symptoms caused by this poisoning very much resembled the symptoms that could be treated by the medicine. He still remembered how he felt when he was ill himself. A second experimental poisoning produced the same results and when he repeated the experiment on friends who agreed to be volunteers, the same or very similar symptoms appeared.

This is not very noteworthy because it is quite common that poisoning by a substance produces very similar results in different individuals. It was the similarity between the symptoms produced during this poisoning and the symptoms for which this substance was effective as a medicine that attracted Hahnemann's attention.

He then tried other medicines on himself and his volunteer experimentees with the same results; the symptoms of poisoning resemble the symptoms that could be treated by the substance.

This was the rediscovery of an old medical principle that says that like can cure like. There is ample historic evidence that other physicists had already used (and were using) this same principle to treat patients successfully. 'Like can cure like' is part of many medical traditions throughout human history.

What then was so special about Hahnemann?

He advocated the use of his experiments as a standard for research on medicines: before a substance/medicine could be used on a patient it should be tested on healthy people. This was in his opinion the only scientific way to acquire knowledge of substances. Testing would allow the medical profession to discover the true indication of various substances that may be used for treating patients. The use of medicines would become scientific and not based on assumptions and habits.

Thus began a period of exhaustive testing of medicines and other substances by Hahnemann and later by his followers, and that is still continuing. It was his opinion that the more substances he tested the more likely he would have a medicine to treat each particular (individual) illness.

Secondly, he was not satisfied with any results. He wanted the tested medicines to be used effectively and without causing side effects to the patient. When he started discovering the efficiency of his tested medicines, he spent all of his energy trying to improve his prescriptions to achieve rapid, smooth and lasting results with his patients. He could not accept that patients' illnesses reappeared after a length of time. He wanted his patients to be cured in the real sense of the word: relieved of their disease and exempt from a relapse of the disease or replacement of the disease by another. He wanted them to be healthier than before he was called out to them. This produced the homeopathic prescription technique that aims at achieving the best possible results for each patient.

From the beginning of his experimenting there was a double problem. Many of the substances Hahnemann had tested or wanted to test were unpleasant to use or even toxic or dangerous and, at the same time, Hahnemann was looking to use medicines causing the least possible side effects or discomfort to the patient. He tried to solve this by using smaller and smaller amounts of substance. He reduced the doses that were used in his experiments more and more and discovered that the very unpleasant and dangerous toxic effects disappeared but that medicines were still effective. The medicines were not only still active but by diluting them they acquired new properties. It was the discovery of these new properties that allowed the birth of homeopathy. Dilution became an important feature of testing, and soon also, in using the medicines.

These new properties of remedies are their capacity to trigger changes in patients who are specifically sensitive to certain remedies.

Such specific sensitivity produces changes in the physical and psychological reactivity of patients or medicine testers after taking high diluted substances. During provings (i.e. medicine testing with high diluted remedies) testers regularly reported original sensations and changes in their attitude to things. Testing these diluted medicines delivered a significant number of symptoms which nobody had ever noticed because they were overshadowed by usual toxic effects experienced at normal doses.

Some testers also reported the unexpected disappearance of longstanding smaller or bigger complaints.

In the beginning, Hahnemann used all sorts of dilutions of medicines but when he realised the importance of diluting, he decided that standardisation was necessary and therefore developed a simple system that allowed him to make very diluted substances without the need for accurate measuring devices. This was done through step-by-step diluting. Each step had a number representing the degree of dilution of the substance (more on his dilution technique in another chapter). The type of dilution used could therefore be recorded with precision and communicated to others.

There were two important aspects of Hahnemann's testing procedure that made his experiments differ from those which others had carried out before him.

1) He accurately recorded all the details of the information he obtained in the exact way the medicine testers expressed them: he used their words and did not make any attempts to 'translate' into medical terms. Such 'translation' would change the value or originality of the obtained information.

2) He did not try to classify this information because that would cause the loss of many details each tester added and therefore the loss of variation in the information. He considered that not only what symptom the tester expressed, but also how he expressed it, was important.

This was a consequence of Hahnemann's principle to respect the individual patient. All the small varieties in the symptoms increased the information he collected. This acted as a guarantee to improving the chance of finding an appropriate remedy for each individual patient.

Others like Sydenham (1624-1689) and Bossier de Sauvages (1707-1793) already expressed the importance of individuality in medicine and the necessity to observe every detail in the patient before him.

ALL symptoms obtained during testing were considered important; both physical and mental symptoms. Hahnemann did not want to explain disease or classify patients' diseases, therefore no symptoms were discarded as being unhelpful or not interesting enough or not fitting some set rules, logic, rationale or symptom classification. All changes perceived by the tester after taking a diluted test substance were recorded in detail in the way they presented themselves. Pains, various sensations, mood changes, dreams, as well as all physical symptoms were treated as part of the reaction of a tester to the substances.

This created a large amount of very difficult-to-use information but at the same time enough material to have a chance to find a solution for each particular case. Although it was a painstaking method to use, Hahnemann insisted that it was a necessity and that such detail would offer the largest variety of patients the best chance of receiving an appropriate remedy.

The richness of the information accumulated over the years still allows homeopaths to discover new facets about existing remedies every day. At the same time it also discourages many from proceeding with a thorough study of homeopathic medicine.

While his experimentation with new medicines was going on, Hahnemann tried to use his newly gained information on patients. He applied the concept that the symptoms produced by a substance during testing were indicators to the use of the substance in a patient showing the same symptoms (like cures like). Very soon he obtained good results and learned little by little how best to use his 'new' medicines on patients.

The first impressive results were obtained during outbreaks of cholera and typhoid fever. In the beginning, it was mainly for such acute (and severe) illnesses that Hahnemann's new remedies proved very effective. This publicity assured a keen interest from fellow physicists. Many joined in the work of developing this infant medicine. Homeopathy then spread throughout Europe and later throughout the world.

Hahnemann tries to improve his prescriptions.

When patients were observed over a longer period than just their acute illness, Hahnemann found that some symptoms that were relieved with his new remedies had a tendency to come back and that often very chronic symptoms were difficult to eliminate. Due to the fact that Hahnemann continued to search for the best way to be effective with these chronic appearances, the elementary homeopathic principles emerged little by little.

His ideal was that:

a) A patient should improve promptly and smoothly (without side effects) to a better state of health after the administration of a remedy and that this should apply not only to the original complaint but also to the patient overall. (It is important to bear this in mind when talking about 'healing crisis' which should not be seen as a necessity for efficient cures!)

b) Additionally, the patient should stay better for a long period of time.

A patient with all his complaints and sufferings is an individual with an original combination of symptoms. This combination of symptoms is the signal to the outside (and patient) that something is going wrong with him and these symptoms can be used to find a cure for the patient. When, by using his new remedies, Hahnemann discovered that he could relieve patients from a few to several and sometimes all their symptoms/sufferings, he concluded that by improving his technique he should be able to help more patients and a larger selection of complaints/symptoms.

Hahnemann wasn't trying to explain disease. He wasn't trying to classify patients according to their symptoms. He did not want to put theoretical limits on what was possible to achieve or tell patients that they could not be helped if they had certain conditions; he was searching for an efficient way to use medicines. He was convinced that if these new remedies were able to reduce symptoms in acute and often severe illnesses, there must be a way to make the prescriptions more accurate to reduce even more symptoms in a patient and be efficient also in chronic and reoccurring illnesses.

During this continuous effort to improve his prescriptions and observations, Hahnemann discovered little by little what was important in selecting remedies:

'Not any type of resemblance between the patient's symptoms and substance's experimental symptoms can be used to procure a homeopathic cure. The resemblance has to be 'homeopathic' to achieve the best possible result.'

The meaning of 'homeopathic resemblance' will be explained in a further chapter. It refers to the fact that homeopathy is more than just any form of 'like cures like'.

By accident, Hahnemann discovered another important characteristic of his remedies. When he made his successive dilutions, in order to assure a homogenous mixture, he used to shake his preparations energetically. During his visits to patients in the countryside, he observed that his liquid remedies were more active in the evening than in the morning. Patients tended to react more to them when he used them at the end of a day's work. The only difference between morning and evening was the shaking his medicine box underwent when travelling on horseback! That is how Hahnemann realised that the shaking or mixing of his medicines during their step-by-step preparation method was important to release the activity of his medicines. This process is called dynamisation.

It is very likely that without Hahnemann's dilution method, homeopathy would never have existed in the way it exists now.

> Note: The following observation has been made by a few of my clients: when in acute cases the prescribed remedy was dissolved in water and vigorously shaken before administration, an immediate reaction to the remedy was often more visible than when a few tablets were left to dissolve in the mouth. This doesn't mean that this method of administering remedies will make a difference in the outcome of the treatment, it gives the impression of 'more energetic action'. It is more homeopathic not to want the patient to react too violently to a remedy. Cures are often more spectacular in the long run when nothing seems to happen.

Little by little Hahnemann discovered how diluted medicines needed to be used in order to achieve the best possible and lasting results and to bring prompt and smooth relief to the patient. His desire for excellence in the treatment of patients together with his vast knowledge of past and present medical thinking and meticulous recordings made it possible to propose and define the principles of homeopathy that are still used today.

The genius of Hahnemann is in the synthesis of centuries of medical thinking combined with rigorous experimenting. This has given rise to a new and original concept on how to treat disease. This new concept also offers a most reliable guideline on how to interpret the results from the administration of (homeopathic) medicines in order to understand what the next best step will be and how well the patient reacted to a remedy.

Today these same principles are still the driving force behind successful homeopathic practice.

Hahnemann's intelligence, knowledge and stubbornness brought him both friends and foes. His ever-increasing criticism of the official medical establishment who at first admired his work, forced him later to move repeatedly to various towns in Europe. He finished his last years in Paris, enjoying a successful homeopathy practice.

Homeopathy was rapidly exported to the American continent where it enjoyed high popularity and success in the 19th century and to the Indian sub-continent where homeopathy is nowadays very widely practised.

Its high popularity in the 19th century throughout Europe and the American continent gave rise to the establishment of homeopathic hospitals and universities. When at the end of this century and the beginning of the 20th century these establishments were annexed to the official hospitals and universities, there followed a rapid decline of homeopathic medicine.

There is a chance that if in our modern times homeopathy tries to win itself recognition by incorporating itself into conventional science that the same may happen again. It is absolutely essential that homeopathy keeps its own education and philosophy if it wants to continue and flourish. This should not be a reason for homeopaths to condemn conventional medicine. Both techniques have their advantages and disadvantages that the medical practitioner should recognise and use to the benefit of the patient.

The Organon.

The Organon is the manuscript in which Hahnemann writes about his knowledge and opinions on medical practice. He describes his concept of acute and chronic illness and details the principles that need to be applied when practising homeopathy.

It is essential to read and study this work thoroughly when training in homeopathic prescription. It is not a recipe book, it doesn't tell you which remedy to use in which case and it is very cumbersome to read.

What it does is to explain clearly what the practitioner's attitude to the patient and his disease must be. It explains how to use the information gathered from the medical experiments to choose the best possible remedy for a particular case and how to evaluate the change in the patient to decide on further treatment.

Without going into a deep study of this book, the following are a few general outlines of the contents of the Organon.

1) Hahnemann puts great emphasis on the observation of the whole patient. The practitioner should use all his senses to obtain as much information as possible from the patient without influencing the patient. This needs to be done in order to understand what needs to be cured in the patient. By this he means that it is necessary to understand what the important symptoms are that individualise the patient: i.e. what is specific to the patient that makes him an individual case. Finding out what needs to be cured does not refer to the conventional diagnosis or the main complaint, it is about pinpointing the symptoms that are specific to the patient and reflect the dynamics of his unhealthy status. These are the symptoms that will guide the homeopath to the best possible prescription.

2) Illness is a deregulation of the 'vital principle'. The 'vital principle' is that which makes the collection of water and other molecules that form our body matter function into one individual. When there is a deregulation of this 'vital principle', disease will show through both physical and mental symptoms in the patient. All the patient's symptoms belong to the disease even when there is no explanation for their connection.

3) The importance of medicine is not to understand or explain what is happening to the patient but to find the best possible cure for the patient.

4) He sets out the conditions that rule the homeopathic testing of new substances.

5) As an explanation of the activity of his medicines he proposes that they act by removing the dynamic (natural) dysfunctioning of the vital principle. The homeopathic remedy generates a similar (artificial) dysfunctioning of the vital principle that eradicates the natural one. After this, the artificial disease recedes when the poisoning effect of the medicine stops, leaving the patient without his previous illness.

6) He stresses the importance of curing without side effects or suffering to the patient.

7) A large part of the manuscript is reserved for the definition and the description of his perception of chronic disease. Hahnemann describes and tries to explain how certain chronic and recurring symptoms are difficult to influence with homeopathic prescriptions. He is dissatisfied with the results he obtains. There is no reason why it cannot be possible to act efficiently on these symptoms using homeopathic remedies. This research and reflection may serve as explanation for the difficulty of the treatment in chronic cases, it is also an attempt to find ways of making prescriptions more effective, an effort that is still going on today.

8) According to his principles, only one remedy should be used at a time and repeated or replaced only when the patient symptoms show that it is necessary. This is the principle of the minimum dose that is the safeguard which prevents any side effects from the use of his new medicines.

The homeopathic principle.

The homeopathic principle is based on a very simple concept; the patient is an individual who can be cured by the remedy that can create a condition similar to his disease. This remedy should be administered in a minimum (i.e. diluted and single) dose.

When we take a deeper look into this concept it will become obvious that the application of this principle will require some skill.

The patient is treated as an individual; when referring to his disease in homeopathy, we don't refer to what we conventionally call the diagnosis. His 'homeopathic disease' is what is characteristic in the patient's present and past symptoms that are an illustration of the dynamic behind the appearance and disappearance of his symptoms and sufferings and the way the patient perceives his suffering and his surroundings. It is about how the malfunctioning of an individual affects the whole of his body including his mind and expresses itself in the form of disease. In short, this means that every patient has his own way of developing AND perceiving disease/symptoms/suffering.

In conventional medicine, it is essential to name the disease before treatment. Homeopathy does not put its effort into the naming of this 'homeopathic disease'. It puts its effort into finding the few (or many) symptoms that are characteristic of the individual patient and therefore characteristic of his personal 'disease'.

These are mostly the uncommon or peculiar symptoms, the symptoms or combination of symptoms that are specific to the patient and are different from what is generally encountered. The patient's conventional diagnosis can in some cases be regarded as a symptom useful to define what is peculiar in the patient but it is never the starting point or sole basis for a homeopathic prescription. Once the 'homeopathic symptoms' have been determined, they will be used to select the best possible homeopathic remedy for the patient.

A homeopathic prescription is not made to treat the patient's disease as named through the conventional diagnosis, it is made to treat the patient with his disease; i.e. there are no homeopathic prescriptions for diseases, prescriptions should be tailor-made for the patient.

Another way to explain the importance of the 'homeopathic' or peculiar symptoms is that they reflect the patient's particular sensitivity. This allows for the choice of the appropriate remedy that will be able to act on the patients 'particular' sensitivity to trigger a healing reaction.

The purpose is not to stimulate the immune system or eliminate toxins. The concept is to imitate the patient's disease in the most perfect way. By doing so the homeopathic remedy will 'wipe out' a part or the whole of the patient's symptoms depending on the degree of similarity between the remedy's dynamic action on the patient and the dynamic affection of the patient.

> Note: The dynamic affection of the patient refers to what can affect the patient, what can trigger off the start of disease in the patient, and the way in which the patient reacts: how the disease establishes itself, how the disease evolves in the patient and what symptoms will present themselves and how one type of disease may be replaced by a different one. The original way in which this happens in one particular patient is the dynamic affection of this particular patient. In homeopathy, disease is seen more like a 'story' that happens to the patient. It is not something static with a name that is present in the patient.
>
> The remedy will be selected for the patient because it is expected to trigger off a similar original evolution/reaction in the patient after administration. This is the dynamic action of the remedy on the patient.
>
> Note: The terms 'stimulation of the immune system' and 'elimination of toxins' describe what can be observed when patients get better; they should never be the aim of the homeopath. They are abstract concepts that describe what seems to happen. We use them because we like to explain the action of a medicine. Nobody can really explain what

these concepts exactly mean although they sound very accurate. Explaining the action of a remedy belongs to the modern medical concept and not to homeopathy.

At first glance, many patients seem to have very comparable affections. They suffer from diarrhoea, headache, flu, depression, cancer, eczema, asthma, anxieties, etc. The closer we look at patients, the more we find differences between patients. Therefore, the closer we look the more individual each patient becomes and the more specific the selection of the remedy can be. The more specific the prescription is for the patient the more efficient the prescription will be. This is the reason why a homeopath needs more time per patient before he can make an adequate prescription. He/she needs to allow the important symptoms to 'rise to the surface' by giving the patient/client the time and circumstances in which this can happen.

To use a concept of our time, let's imagine that the 'well-selected' remedy contains the information that the patient can use to remedy the dysfunction of their body-and-mind entity. The more this information is adapted to the patient, the better the results will be. To accept this vision on health and disease it is important to accept that a living creature is more than the sum of his molecules and chemical reactions. We are not robots made of different body parts; we have to accept that there is something in us (the vital principle, energy, soul, whatever you want to call it) that organises the coherence between all the materials that make up our body.

> Note 1: On the subject of what makes us, there are three possible visions. We could have an all-material vision, considering that only the things we can measure really exist. We could have an all-energy vision, considering that our body is only the expression of some form of energy that creates an image in our minds. Thirdly, we can accept that material exists and that there is some form of energy that governs it. In the case of our body, Hahnemann called the energy that governs the body the Vital Principle.

Note 2: Our modern view on the brain controlling the body like in a machine is not accurate. Already Spinoza stressed the importance of seeing the body as a unity of mind and matter. There is no dualism of mind and body as Descartes and his followers wanted it to be. Modern biology has proven this many times over in the last few years. Benjamin Libet, a neurophysiologist, showed this through one of his experiments. For medical reasons in certain cases of brain surgery the patient is kept conscious (the brain is not sensitive to pain). A few of his patients were willing to participate in the following test: he asked them to raise their arm while he measured the electrical activity in the part of the brain that 'consciously commands' this movement. Every time, the start of the movement of the arm preceded the start of the electrical activity by approximately 300 milliseconds. As a consequence one can decide to raise one's arm but the decision (action in the brain) is not the cause of action. The decision and the movement are one; they are just two different aspects of the action. Mind and body are one. This experiment has been confirmed by many others and has been extended to the physical aspects of emotions; an emotion takes place at the same time in our body as in our mind, they are just two different ways of expressing an emotions: it is very common to feel one's emotions in the abdomen.

This is the reason that we should be careful with our definition of, and views on, psychosomatic disease; both the psychological problem and the physical problem belong to the patient. The behaviour, anxiety or other psychological symptoms in the patient are just other aspects of 'their disease'. They are symptoms just like physical symptoms. Psychosomatic diseases only indicate a certain sensitivity in the patient.

Of course this does not accommodate our desire to explain and classify things.

Note 3: The genome project that promises us future miracles in medicine is fascinating but forgets one thing; we are not our chromosomes. We are the result of a constant interaction between our chromosomes and our surroundings. The surroundings determine the expression of our chromosomes and the expression of our chromosomes determine how we (and our chromosomes) react to the surroundings. The fixing of a chromosome will have an influence on our health but this influence may differ greatly from individual to individual. One potential benefit of this research may very well be the future acknowledgement by science that homeopathy has always been right in pressing that the patient should be seen and treated as an individual.

After having selected the symptoms that make the patient an individual, it is now time to find the best possible remedy that will have a healing action on the patient.

Like cures like: we need to find the remedy that 'resembles' the patient in the expression of his 'disease'. This means that if the remedy was given to the patient when he is healthy he would develop a very similar condition.

To do this, a comparable exercise needs to be carried out regarding the remedies as is carried out regarding the patient. We have to study the symptoms that are produced by the different remedies, when they were tested on healthy persons, in such a way that we develop a picture or understanding of each remedy. It is necessary to search through the information available on each remedy to find what makes the remedy peculiar, what is specific/individual to the remedy, what does its specific and original dynamic effect look like. We have to create disease pictures for remedies that help us in remembering and understanding how a remedy may affect the patient.

To create a 'remedy disease picture', it is important to use the uncommon, peculiar or very typical symptoms associated with the remedy.

The information we have at our disposal to study the effects of a given substance when ingested, comes from

1) The tests on healthy people (provings)

2) Accidental intoxication reports.

3) Healing activity of substances when administered to patients: i.e. symptoms that have disappeared in a patient after the use of a remedy.

The study of remedies is done by using this information in order to establish what are the special (homeopathic) symptoms belonging to each remedy to create dynamic disease pictures of remedies. This is of great help in the selection of the appropriate remedy for each patient when often several remedies seem to be indicated.

When we take a close look at the accumulation of symptom information of each remedy, this will lead to two observations:

1) There are many remedies that have many symptoms in common. General symptoms such as cough, headache, diarrhoea, etc are common symptoms that are shared by a very large number of remedies and are therefore not very helpful in the process of remedy selection. When the patient's complaint is one of these common symptoms, it is important to search for other clues (symptoms), which will narrow down the possible remedies that seem indicated in his case.

2) Over the years, through experience, it has become clear that certain remedies have a particular 'reliable' effect on specific symptoms, syndromes or body functions. Over the years these

observations have been recorded with, as a consequence, a tendency for 'reflex' prescription of these remedies for the symptoms or syndromes for which their efficiency seemed to be reliable. For instance Belladonna is said to be a remedy for fever, Rhus tox a remedy for rheumatism, Arsenicum album a remedy for diarrhoea. Instead of doing a proper homeopathic assessment of all the patient's symptoms before remedy selection, and base this selection on the symptoms that are thought to have a homeopathic value, remedies are selected following the conventional diagnosis (i.e. name of the disease) of the patient. This technique is for many a more attractive way of using homeopathic medicines. Through their renowned efficiency certain remedies developed popular use in certain conditions.

In homeopathy one can never say that for a particular condition there exists a particular remedy. The remedy selection needs to be based on the particulars of the patient, his condition being one of the factors that may influence the choice of the remedy. Also, the testing of remedies is never pushed up to the situation of producing disease; this would not be very ethical. Therefore the capacity for producing a specific disease is not known for many homeopathic remedies. Associations between remedies and diseases come from experience with the uses of these remedies; this is called reputable action. Ideally the selection of a remedy should be based on other symptoms than pure physical/disease symptoms. This will ensure a much more 'homeopathic' prescription.

> Note: It is not always essential to have a perfect 'understanding' of the activity of a remedy to use it in a homeopathic way. If the right homeopathic symptom(s) are selected they will direct the homeopath to the most appropriate remedy by using a homeopathic repertory. That is one of the strengths of homeopathy; it is possible to use very unusual medicines successfully through application of the homeopathic principle without the need of knowing or understanding such medicines. This gives the individual patient a better chance. There are many

successful case records where patients have benefited a great deal from remedies the practitioner had never used before and of which he had no knowledge.

Starting from the simple principle of homeopathy, it now has become clear that the practitioner needs to excel in the art of case taking. He needs the skill to spot the patient's specific or homeopathic symptoms that will guide him to the best possible remedy. To choose the best possible remedy, he also needs to be able to know or find out what is important in the remedy he wants to use and, thirdly, he needs to understand what the nature of the resemblance must be between the remedy and the patient to achieve a homeopathic cure.

The 'scientific' character of homeopathy is the experimentation with drugs on healthy people before their use on patients. The prescription of the right remedy needs training and skill, which sometimes takes more the form of Art rather than a pure application of set rules.

When one wants to obtain the full potential from a homeopathic prescription it is important to set aside conventional/scientific/reasoning in order to let the patient 'speak' and give away what is homeopathically important in his case without interfering with scientific prejudice.

It is not always necessary to go into lengthy consultations to obtain the information that leads the practitioner to a good prescription. Also, prescriptions don't always need to be 'perfectly' homeopathic to achieve results.

It is even possible to obtain good or acceptable results when prescribing remedies on a syndrome or symptom without making the prescription fit the individual like a glove, through a 'perfect' homeopathic attitude.

What is important to remember is that the more efficient a remedy needs (or is wished) to be, the more accurate the homeopathic principles need to be applied.

Using homeopathy.

Is it really so important to go into such detail about 'pure' homeopathy? One could argue that this is all irrelevant theorising and purist thoughts when patients can benefit from the use of homeopathically prepared remedies given to them in various other ways and combinations.

Even Hahnemann who had established the very precise homeopathic principles did not always apply them to the letter. There is evidence that at some point he tried all sorts of successions of remedies and facilitated prescription methods. This was because Hahnemann was still learning and experimenting with his new technique in order to become more efficient in using his new medicines. He never discarded any experiment out of pure principle; his purpose was to serve the patient and not his homeopathic doctrine. The end conclusion he made after each of the trials that deviated from the pure homeopathic principles, was that these alternatives did not offer the same benefits to the patient as his original method of the use of a singular remedy specially selected for the patient.

In a similar search for 'easier' uses of homeopathically prepared remedies, many of his followers devised 'alternative' methods of selection and prescription. New ideas have a tendency to appear and then disappear again. The introduction of new ideas may help homeopathic medicine to grow up and increase its possibilities as long as practitioners concentrate on the benefit for the patient rather than their own benefit. There are, nowadays, a variety of teachings throughout the world, all classifying themselves under the name of homeopathy. Some are more true to homeopathic principles than others.

'To make the homeopathic prescriptions easier and more reliable' is a driving force behind several variations on the homeopathic principle. Making an efficient and rapid acting homeopathic prescription is not always straightforward. Sometimes (often) it is difficult to find those symptoms that make a patient an individual. Also, one can never be sure whether the prescription is going to have the expected result. These difficulties are the driving force behind the continuing search for simpler, easier or more 'reliable' ways to select and use homeopathically prepared remedies.

> Note: A medicine is homeopathically prepared when diluted according to Hahnemann's technique. It is homeopathic if it produces a smooth, rapid, efficient and lasting healing action on a patient following the administration of a minute dose.

The practice of empiric medicine where observation and selection of a remedy is made without using 'scientific reasoning or logic' is something that does not come easily. We like to have logic or common sense explanations for what we do, whether this explanation is scientific or whether this explanation suits a particular vision on health and disease. This helps to give us a secure feeling about the decisions we make and this fits in with the way we perceive things.

Many alternative homeopathic prescription techniques have some kind of a reasoning process built in to them extracted from modern medical science that gives the impression of more secure or logical prescriptions which gives assurance to the practitioner and client/patient.

Another factor that influenced variations on the homeopathic theme is the cultural differences and communication difficulties between various homeopathy groups in different countries. Better communication nowadays is bringing homeopaths together making room for lively exchanges. There will always be differences in the practice of homeopathy due to the sensitivity of each individual but generally the consensus seems to orientate towards the original principles as Hahnemann laid them out.

Also, it is not everybody's desire, need or conviction to obtain a perfect homeopathic cure: e.g. to get a rapid response that has a profound and long lasting effect on the entire patient with the use of a minimum amount of medicine. The severity of the case or the type of illness that is present in the patient, the kind of service the client/patient is looking for, the effort the patient/client wants to put into the search for the best possible prescription, the kind of information that is obtained from and about the patient all come into the calculation when a prescription strategy is decided upon.

Whether homeopathy is sought for the treatment of a long-standing mental illness in a person, a skin problem in a dog or a cough in a group of fattening pigs, the same homeopathic principles apply but the approach may be different.

As a general rule: the more chronic, insidious and severe the illness is, the more precise the prescription needs to be to obtain good results. Acute, small day-to-day complaints react most of the time quite well to the standard recipes or a rapidly selected remedy out of a small group. Remember that many acute conditions/symptoms disappear by themselves regardless of any treatment given.

When the ailment becomes chronic or repetitive, when organ tissues have undergone considerable damage (heart failure, arthritis), when the patient's mood is starting to suffer (depression), when there are longstanding allergic or auto-immune conditions (skin, rheumatoid arthritis, asthma, etc) and when tumours or cancers are involved, remedy selection will need to be very precise to obtain appreciable results. These results can go from improvement in the patient's quality of life to sometimes very impressive cures.

The nature of the complaint and the result that is required will therefore play an important role in the attitude of the homeopath.

The quality of conventional medicine is improving very rapidly. Considerable efforts are made to eliminate side effects from treatments as much as possible. For several important conditions like hormonal imbalances, some tumours and cancers, life threatening conditions, infections and other emergencies there are very convenient treatments. There is no harm in using them while looking for a homeopathic complementary treatment that, if it proves sufficiently efficient, will diminish and sometimes replace conventional treatments. Many people who have felt or seen the benefit of a good homeopathic prescription will confirm that homeopathy can in these cases offer increased quality and duration of life and result frequently in a substantial reduction in use of conventional medicines. Spectacular cures also happen, if homeopathy/homeopath is given the chance. It all comes down to how good the selection of the remedy was for the patient.

When homeopathy is used alongside (heavy) medication, homeopathic prescriptions need to be more accurate than usual to be able to have a homeopathic effect on the patient because of the interfering presence/action of such conventional medicines. A well-trained and honest homeopath should over time be able in most cases to see the difference between the activity of the conventional treatment and the activity of his homeopathic prescription.

At the same time it is not always necessary to use modern chemicals in day-to-day treatments. With a little motivation and a little patience, applying homeopathy as a first choice can be very rewarding, keeping conventional medicine ready if necessary. Everyday homeopathic medicine produces very satisfying little wonders of beautiful, smaller and bigger cures Persistently eliminating disturbing symptoms by using conventional drugs is often not very beneficial to the long-term health of the patient.

What is classical homeopathy?

Classical homeopathy refers to the use of one remedy at a time, selected through the application of original homeopathic principles for the individual patient. Each case will be approached individually with the intention of achieving the best possible results in the shortest space of time. There will be no peeling of the onion idea, no pre-established succession of remedies, no prescription based on conventional diagnosis. Only the homeopathic symptoms of the patient guide the classical homeopath to his prescription. The advantage of this system is that over time cases never become blurred, it is always clear what the homeopathic attitude to the case should be. This strategy also gives the best chances of finding the best possible remedy that will bring the patient to a healthier mind and body situation compared to that before the motivation of the consultation.

Classical homeopathy can be easily distinguished from pluralistic and complexist homeopathy:

-Pluralistic homeopathy will use one or more remedies in a more or less quick succession. Prescriptions are often syndrome or diagnosis orientated. The advantage is the possibility of making rapid prescriptions. Pluralistic homeopathy resembles conventional practice. Remedies are selected for the patient based on their renowned activity. The disadvantage is that over time cases often become confused and no real progress in the patient's health state is made. This is a complaint that is often made by homeopaths who after a few years of pluralistic practice discover classical homeopathy.

-Complexist homeopathy makes use of mixtures of homeopathic remedies. These mixtures may be commercially prepared or more or less custom made. Various theories have emerged justifying the mixing of homeopathic medicines. Some mixtures are the result of experience.
When several homeopathic substances are mixed together (or given on the same day), a 'new' homeopathic medicine has been created. The activity of a mixture of homeopathic medicines does not represent the sum of its ingredients; it is a new medicine that needs a proving (i.e. homeopathic testing on healthy people) to discover its proper homeopathic indications. The homeopathic principle is not applied but some mixtures achieve appreciable results based on the experience by practitioners. Results are symptom driven and do not achieve real lasting homeopathic improvements. It is not advisable to use these complexes on severe diseases.

The successful use of complexist homeopathic preparations is based on experience and not on the application of the homeopathic principles.

Note: An example of different approaches using homeopathic medicines

Homeopathy is requested for a dog with skin problems. Despite an efficient flea therapy there is a constant flea allergy type skin condition causing regular flare-ups with lots of scratching on the back causing patches with skin infection. The dog is agitated when he scratches and then also drinks more often. There are a few warts around his neck and head and recently an arthritic lesion has been diagnosed on his left shoulder.

The classical homeopath would have listened a while to what the owners had to say about their dog and, after having examined him, observed his behaviour in the consultation room. The dog hates to be approached by strangers, he makes regular attempts to escape from the owner's garden and in the consultation room the vet observes that he has a strange spasm of his left upper lip from time to time. Cuprum metallicum is given once in a 200K dose. The behaviour of the dog improves, the arthritis disappears followed by the disappearance of the skin problems and warts in one month. A slight relapse of the skin problems three months later is quickly controlled with a further dose of Cuprum metallicum.

A Pluralist homeopath may set up the following treatment: One dose of Sulfur as a start to 'clean up' the dog's skin. Then a dose of Arsenicum album once per day 5 days per week for a month because of his agitation. A dose of diluted Flea Saliva in 30C once per week to diminish the allergic reaction and Rhus tox once per day in the morning to treat the arthritis.

If the dog improves, it will be difficult to know what remedy achieved what result. What would the attitude be if the symptoms disappear to come back next year? Very often the same treatment will not work again.

A complexist treatment may be as follows:
A mixture of, Arsenicum album, Juglans cinirea, Echinacea, Lycopodium, Sepia can be used twice daily for three weeks. A different complex may be used to treat the arthritic problem.

Classical homeopathy is the most logic homeopathic technique for the following reasons:

- Once we accept the principle of similitude as a healing method, classical prescription is the only intellectually acceptable technique. The patient is   one; you can't just cut them into pieces for the convenience of prescription.
- The advantage of the system is that the practitioner does not need to have a perfect knowledge of each remedy he or she wants to use. The technique allows for finding successful unusual remedies.
- There is more room for the use of complete Material Medica's to verify a remedy for the patient: in classical homeopathy the large amount of information gathered on each tested remedy can become useful.

The case records in the second part of this book will give you ample examples of these observations.

Individual medicine?

Earlier, there was an allusion to treating a group of fattening pigs. Do we then have to find a homeopathic medicine for each and every animal when homeopathy is sought to treat such a group of animals? This would be very impracticable if the group contains tens or hundreds of individuals.

The answer is no. The homeopathic individualisation in such a case where a large number of individuals need treating at the same time is directed towards the group that expresses a temporary disease. This disease can be a cough, a fever, or dysentery. Such a disease is a collective disease. It is what individualises the particular passage of cough; the other symptoms like the type of cough, time of aggravation, any behaviour changes in the group during the disease, circumstances of appearance of the disease that accompanies the cough will determine what the homeopathic remedy will be for the group's disease.

In these cases the homeopath will look for what is peculiar to the passage of the disease in the group. Such a group can be a group of calves housed together, a building containing 10,000 poultry, a racehorse yard, a class of pupils, the inhabitants of a geographical part of a country.

What these groups have in common is that they are all under the influence of very similar external factors. When a transmittable disease appears, the expression of this disease in the group will be very much determined by the circumstances in which the group lives, like climate, weather, season, type of building, common stress situation, similar feeding pattern, air pollution, relation to keeper or government etc,.

It is common for classical human homeopaths living in the same region to link up to exchange prescription information when there is an epidemic like a winter flu outbreak. This enables them to rapidly establish which remedy will be most effective on most patients during the epidemic.

Hahnemann first used this idea when he determined the remedy that proved to cure most patients (90%) during each dysentery or cholera outbreak he was confronted with. The remedy was selected by determining the particular symptoms that accompanied the classical cholera or dysentery symptoms like a certain type of skin rash, whether the patients were more or less agitated, whether the patients where thirsty or not, how fast disease set in, when disease set in, etc,.

It is not the patient but the recognisable transmittable disease that affects a group or a geographical region that will be individualised to select the homeopathic remedy that will be effective for most individuals in the group. There will always be a small proportion (5 - 10%) in the group that will not respond to the common remedy. These patients will need an individualised prescription.

Chronic common conditions will not be suited for this approach. For instance asthma outbreaks in the spring are a common expression of a common disease that needs a different approach for each patient! Asthma is not caused by pollen. Pollen is a common stress factor but more personal factors are needed to 'allow' asthma to develop. Every patient has its own typical asthma disease that needs its own specific treatment; asthma does not spread like a recognisable infectious disease.

Epidemics like AIDS, that thrive in certain well-defined geographical regions, and therefore act like real epidemics, may well be very efficiently tackled by a common remedy within the recognised region. Finding such a remedy is not an easy task. This will be less likely in the western world where the common factors for the AIDS epidemic are more difficult to identify. It will be more useful to treat the disease as an individual disease.

What to tell the homeopath?

This is a very simple question to answer: tell him what you think, what your feelings are about the/your case. Don't try and tell the practitioner what you think he wants to know. The purpose of the consultation is not to please the homeopath with your answers but to create an atmosphere where useful 'homeopathic' information about the patient emerges that can be used to select the best possible remedy. Don't be afraid to say strange things; the purpose is not to hold a scientific exchange with the homeopath. Any information may be useful; often the strangest things are the most helpful in finding an appropriate remedy. It is important to be spontaneous; say the things the way they come into your head without trying to be 'relevant' or 'scientific'.

Exchanges between homeopath and client/patient should be free from bias. Both patient and third party observers can be used to increase information.

If you are the patient, the homeopath will be specially interested in hearing your opinion about things, your feelings and the things that disturb you the most coming from the outside world or yourself.

If your animal (or child) is the patient, tell him what makes the patient special, what are the strange, uncommon or inexplicable things you find about him or her. Often what seem to be completely unrelated symptoms are the keys to very efficient prescriptions.

Much emphasis is put on finding the modalities of the patient (i.e. the things the patient is sensitive to like the weather, food, temperature or time of the day). When such symptoms are obvious they can be very helpful in determining an appropriate remedy. Never should one search for specific symptoms; it is important to let the patient talk about what matters (through a third party in case of children or animals). Allowing time and making effort to observe the patient is what counts. It is not up to the homeopath to determine what is necessary to be able to select an appropriate remedy for the patient, it is the patient who 'decides' what is important.

What about follow-up consultations?

Follow-up consultations are there to assess the improvement in the patient. Just because the original complaint has disappeared does not mean that the patient has been homeopathically improved. The need for the repetition of a remedy or replacement with another remedy is based on the homeopathic principles proposed by Hahnemann. His ideal of improvement of the patient is often beyond what is generally expected by the patient.

The health consumer can use classical homeopathy in two ways. The homeopath can be consulted when there is an (acute) problem that motivates the patient to look for help and as soon the problem disappears no further consultations are requested by the patient. Often the homeopath receives no feed-back and when the patient returns months or years later this is when a new (or the same) motivation for help has sprung up again. This is very much the problem – solution approach that is applied in modern medicine.

It is possible to have a more long-term and therefore proactive approach to homeopathy. Consulting the homeopath after improvement helps in understanding and evaluating the patient. This allows one to decide whether the improvement in the patient went according to the homeopathic rules and whether a repeat or renewal prescription is warranted. Such follow-up helps in ensuring that the patient really improves holistically. This will assure long term benefit and may be more efficient than any type of preventative medicine. It is as if homeopathic medicines can be used as a form of prevention. Using a medicine in a sort of 'preventative manner' does not seem logical according to our usual way of perceiving things. It is also difficult to persuade somebody to consult when their health worries are not foremost in their mind. Consultations need not be weekly or monthly. For people this can be done yearly, in the case of animals this needs to be more than once per year. The shorter life span in our animals makes disease evolve at a faster pace than in humans.

A better way of explaining things would be as follows: the more effort and time that is put into the follow-up of a patient, the more likely it is that an efficient long-term solution will be found. It is often out of little details that successful prescription arises. These details don't always 'happen' at any time. Repeated consultations are a way of increasing the chances of making them happen. In cases where it takes several consultations before the patient finally benefits from good homeopathic prescription it asks much good-will and confidence from the health consumer.

In the end it is up to you to decide what you want and where you want to go. 'Homeopathy, what to expect?' is there to explain the possibilities and the difficulties and to help you in making your choice. It is also important to remember that these explanations only apply to classical homeopathy. Alternative 'natural' therapies that use homeopathic prepared medicines are based on other approaches to medicine and don't always subscribe to the same long-term approach.

Note: A client who very quickly sensed the homeopathic principles asked me to start homeopathic prescription on her dog allowing time to find a suitable remedy for him before anything serious could happen. At the time of the first consultation the dog only had a minor skin problem but it was slowly approaching a respectable age. It was a good move because it took several different prescriptions before a really efficient remedy appeared on the scene. The reason being that the remedy was a rather unusual one.

Homeopathic medicine and homeopathically prepared medicines.

As already mentioned before, there are many variations on the homeopathic principles. We often hear or read about nosodes, pollen, isotherapeutic remedies, cancer remedies, Bach flowers, homeopathic vaccines, antidotes etc., what are they?

In homeopathy practice, prescriptions are based on the symptoms of the patient compared to the symptoms of substances obtained through experimenting on healthy individuals.

Many of the remedies that may be classified under the above names, have never undergone rigorous experimentations. They are the result of reasoning often using a mixture of medical thoughts, ideas and experience (including homeopathic ones). Known substances from medical traditions or newly discovered medical substances are then homeopathically prepared (i.e. diluted). The homeopathic preparation technique will diminish their potential toxic, infectious or other dangerous (or illegal) effects and may enhance some of their beneficial effects. Prescription rules are obtained through reasoning and rely very much on conventional diagnosis.

Through their regular use on patients, practitioners obtain experience with them. Prescription of these remedies belongs then to experience based medicine. One such remedy (Carcinosinum) has over the years acquired a good status as a homeopathic remedy and is now regularly used by classical homeopaths applying the homeopathic principles. This shows the relation of experience-based medicine and homeopathy. If proper records are kept over time with relation to the use of a medicine in experience-based medicine, they can be used later to have a homeopathic look at this medicine and use it for homeopathic prescription where the selection of the remedy is based on the patient's peculiarities.

Because these new remedies are often used as part of more complex prescriptions, no good homeopathic (symptoms) information is available on them, which makes their use in classical homeopathy difficult or unlikely.

The use of the above named techniques cannot be classified as homeopathy. This doesn't mean they cannot be effective. Some produce satisfactory results. The main problem with these systems is that there is no real universal guide on how they should best be applied. They depend very much on individual practitioners' experience and ability and are as such difficult to teach. Their advantage is that their 'indications' are usually easier to understand and accept because they conform to our collective modern rational way of thinking, which makes their use attractive and satisfactory.

Special consideration is needed on the subject of homeopathic vaccines. Much use is made of nosodes to 'vaccinate' animals as an alternative to conventional vaccines.

The bad name gained by vaccinating within the homeopathic world dates mainly from the beginning of vaccines (cowpox etc) and later controversies on vaccines. Earlier vaccines used to have many more side effects than modern vaccines. Stating blandly that vaccinating is bad for you is an unbalanced approach. The major problem with vaccines is that we are not really objectively informed on them. The pharmaceutical industry only releases the information it wants to release. Politics and economic interests have become players in the decision-making on vaccines, causing the subject to be taken away from the guarantee of objective discussion.

There are vaccines that are administered unnecessarily. There are vaccines that have worse side effects than are admitted. There are vaccines that are administered too early in life or too often. Vaccines seem to be the answer to all problems in medicine for which there are no effective treatments or which are conceived to be dangerous. Too much credit is given for the elimination of infectious disease by vaccines. (Much of the improvement in our health and life span is to be attributed to better living conditions rather than to medicine.)

These observations feed the controversy on conventional vaccines and need to be addressed.

Being totally against vaccines is not a good strategy. Vaccines have prevented many (humans and animals alike) from developing dangerous and crippling diseases. Considering vaccines as the only guarantee for good health is not a good strategy either. There is a long open debate needed which we will never obtain as long as all medical organisations benefit too much from direct and indirect funding by the industry and conventional (rational) medicine is seen as the only acceptable answer to medicine.

The point of homeopathic vaccines is that they don't really exist! What is proposed as homeopathic vaccines are homeopathically prepared parts of a vaccine, an infectious agent or elimination caused by an infectious disease. They are called nosodes. The idea that such preparations are active as a preventative or even as a cure for the identified infectious disease comes from the principle of isotherapy.

Isotherapy is based on treating with what 'causes the same'. For instance: to treat flu, a patient may be given the flu virus diluted and prepared according to the homeopathic method. (homeopathy treats with what causes a similar disease picture) In some situations this technique can (and has often been) very effective. To use isotherapy as a preventative is presuming that we know that this technique is going to be the appropriate approach at the time the protection is required (i.e. before the disease strikes) and that we administer the remedy close enough to the occurrence of the infectious disease for it to be effective. This poses a challenge. One should never forget that efficient homeopathic prescription is based on comparison of the peculiar original symptoms of the patient with symptoms attributed to remedies. It is impossible to know with sufficient certainty how the next epidemic disease is going to behave. It will reveal itself with its usual symptoms so we can diagnose it but for efficient homeopathic prescription we will use the unusual symptoms that appear at the same time as the epidemic.

Isotherapy does not make antibodies as a vaccination does; it does something else. This is one of the reasons why these 'medicines' should not be called vaccines. Isotherapeutic medicines have an influence on the patient; how this works in prevention nobody knows. In some well-controlled situations such as farms and kennels, the use of isotherapeutic prevention is more easily justified than for individual patients.

Another troubling aspect is the repetition of administration of these nosodes. How often do they need to be administered to be effective? If we administer them on a regular basis we may cause the effect of a proving on the patient: the (repeated) administration of a homeopathic remedy to a patient can result in the appearance of symptoms in the patient caused by the remedy (i.e. homeopathic intoxication). It should not be forgotten that administering homeopathically diluted remedies may cause symptoms to appear in the subject; this is the way provings of new medicines are performed. We cannot at the same time pretend that homeopathically prepared remedies are harmless and at the same time say that they are effective; this is intellectually not acceptable. Considering this, homeopathic vaccines may be as detrimental to certain sensitive subjects as conventional vaccines.

I have used conventional vaccines on many animals for a long time. I have seen animals becoming unwell after vaccines but these cases are not the rule. Modern vaccines are not without danger but can be very effective if used appropriately and not blindly as it is often the case.

These are just a few points in the discussion on vaccinations. Using nosodes as preventative treatment needs to be justified on a case-by-case base. It cannot be used as an ordinary alternative to conventional vaccines.

Homeopathy and placebo

The relationship between homeopathy and placebo has different aspects.

In scientific medical research, placebo is used to distinguish between the activity of a medicine and an inactive presentation of this medicine. The placebo drug in the trial has the same presentation and make as the medicine without the active ingredient. One group will take the medicine, the other group will take the placebo while both groups spend the time of the study in the same, controlled circumstances. Any difference in the two groups after the trial time can then be attributed to the active ingredient.

This is the modern way to test and provide proof of the activity of medicines.

It is possible to prove that homeopathically prepared substances make a difference between two patient groups by performing such a trial. If one group receives a homeopathically prepared medicine and the other only the dilutant, it can be possible to find differences between the two groups after the trial period and therefore prove that a homeopathic substance can make a difference. 'Making a difference' can in certain cases mean 'having a positive/curing effect' in other cases there is just a difference and nothing more.

It is very difficult to prove that homeopathic remedies can cure/improve the patient (or disease) in this way. To obtain a cure for the patient, a remedy needs to be homeopathic, selected especially for the patient according to his particular symptoms. The control group and the treated group should therefore only contain patients for which the same homeopathic remedy applies. This implies that both groups have to be made up out of very identical individuals, a difficult condition to fulfill. The individuality principle that is the centre of homeopathy is the main obstacle to such types of trials. A remedy is not selected for a specific disease; therefore placebo trials are not the ideal way to prove the effectiveness of homeopathic prescription.

(Effectiveness of homeopathy can be compared between heterogeneous groups when both groups benefitting from conventional medicine but only one group also benefits from homeopathic prescription. In such a trial it is the effectiveness of homeopathic prescription that is proven and not the efficiency of one or another homeopathic remedy.)

The other aspect of placebo is related to the effect the prescription/practitioner has on the patient without the interference of a substance. This placebo effect exists in all types of medicine and is the consequence of a mixture of the following factors: the susceptibility of the patient, the atmosphere of the consultation and the personality of the practitioner. This form of medicine is often referred to as 'healing'.

Note: An English homeopath found that he had better results (satisfied patients) when consulting in a nice wood furnished room and when he dispensed his medicines himself from old fashion bottles containing the remedies in powder form than when he practised in the 'clean' environment of a hospital handing out written prescriptions.

Because in homeopathy there is a more entwined relationship between the client/patient and the practitioner, there is a greater chance for a placebo effect to be caused by the interaction during the consultation than in conventional medicine where consultations are often much shorter and 'down to business'. This is something most homeopaths are aware of and take into account when they make an assessment of the patient's improvement.

Some homeopaths make use of the prescription of placebo in the form of a remedy with a homeopathic name that has no active ingredient, to permit the evaluation of the improvement of their patient. This may help them determining the difference between the placebo effect he has on the patient and the real effect of a prescription at a later (or earlier) date. The purpose is not to cheat but to be able to judge the reaction of a patient in the most appropriate way to determine the best possible prescription strategy without interfering in the evolution of the patient by administering him a diluted remedy.

A common criticism is that homeopathy only acts through placebo effect. It is certainly true that a certain amount of improvements acknowledged by patients is due to the very nature of the homeopathic consultation. I had a case myself where I am sure that part of the spectacular result I obtained on the behaviour of a 5 year old dog was due to the consultation. The owner had talked for more than a half hour about his dog and it was obvious that his attitude to his dog had changed somewhat during the consultation. Dogs are very sensitive to the attitude of the members of their 'family' and in this case the 're-established' relationship between owner and dog' was partly responsible for the dramatic improvement in the dog's behaviour.

As long as the practitioner recognises this phenomenon it can only be of benefit to the patient.

When homeopathic remedies are part of a more spiritual or shamanism type of medicine it becomes even more difficult to determine what part the homeopathic remedy plays in the healing process. There is no harm in this provided that the practitioner uses a critical approach to evaluate and direct his patient and also when we are careful to attribute an improvement to the activity of a remedy.

Three different kinds of practising medicine.

The central premise and concept of modern medicine is to make the best possible effort to understand and explain disease using all the possibilities science gives us. This understanding of the functioning of the body in health and disease is considered to lead to the discovery and rational use of medicines and techniques to bring about a cure by interfering with what has been established/thought to be the cause or the wrong functioning of the patient. Science, measurements, statistics and reasoning are the tools that rule decision-making. Measuring is considered the key to understanding and reliability.

> Note: It is interesting to know that one of the founders of experimental modern medicine in the 19th century (Claude Bernard) also said that by measuring and determining biological processes we reduce the chance of representing reality. He was an advocate of the application of science and mathematics to medicine while he recognised the impossibility of grasping and representing the reality of the biological processes through this method.

The medical establishment oversees the correctness of the experiments and their conclusions to produce the rules for diagnosis and prescription. Medical practitioners are there to apply the established rules (with a tendency of diminishing freedom of choice).

In conventional medicine the establishment of the diagnosis is essential: conventional medicine is diagnosis orientated. During the consultation, the practitioner will search for the symptoms that are typical for a disease. Before starting treatment the patient needs to be 'reduced' to a diagnosis. The consequence of the modern view on medicine is that without a diagnosis treatment cannot be established.

A second aspect of modern medicine is that medical techniques and medicines need to be evaluated for their effectiveness before they can be used. Before a treatment is accepted is has to be proven to be effective. This is called evidence-based medicine. Because all medical trials to determine the appropriate treatment are so controlled, rigorous, checked and revised, this way of working gives the medical community a sense of (false?) security. This sense of security (everything has been scientifically proven) creates a strong foundation for the value of modern medicine. This 'facilitates' the work of conventional health practitioners by reducing their responsibility as long as they work within the established framework. This also establishes a secure feeling with the health consumer and sometimes opens the (flood)gates for litigation?

Because of our western education we consider this logic and accept this system as the only rational way of practising medicine.

This system reduces treatment possibilities because great efforts are necessary to evaluate each treatment for each particular disease; economics play a major role and often reduce much of modern medicine to a commercial activity (drug companies etc)

Another kind of medicine, which represents the majority of medical practice, is experience-based medicine. This is very different from 'experiment-based medicine' (or evidence-based medicine). In experience-based medicine, surgical techniques and use of medicines is guided by previous experiences about their activity/effectiveness by a singular practitioner, a group of practitioners or tradition and popular beliefs. Herbal medicine is a typical example. The results of the use of herbs and other substance over the centuries following a variety of philosophic or accidental circumstances, have been passed on in verbal and written form through generations. There is no set principle or testing method that justifies why such or such a medicine is used. It is the renowned activity of each medicine or technique that motivates prescription or self-medication. Tendencies, conviction and accumulated information rather then a well defined principle, rule or controlled tests are the motives for prescription.

> Note: Nowadays it is easy to access large amounts of information through the Internet. When extensive research is done for herbal medicines, it is common to find that many medicinal plants have the widest possible range of indications. These indications may vary from region to region. If one makes the sum of these indications the list is usually very long, going from local applications for wounds to concoctions for cancers made from the same plant. This is especially true for the most popular of herbal remedies.

Many homeopathic remedies are used for their renowned effects. This tradition refers to experience-based medicine. Results may be acceptable in not too complicated pathologies. This form of medicine is very popular. Treatments are usually accompanied by appealing explanations and philosophies.

There is also a fair amount of conventional practice that can be classified under this type of medicine. It is not uncommon to hear how one or another physicist knows how to treat one or another illness more efficiently then another practitioner due to his 'experience'. Conventional medicine makes continuous efforts to eliminate such 'non-regulated' practice. The private judgment of an individual is less and less appreciated in favour of commonly decided treatment strategies and practice.

Modern medicine should not forget that many conventional treatments that have accepted official recognition after scientific investigating and testing originated from experience based medicine.

The difference of homeopathy compared with the two previous types of medical practice is that homeopathy is a system for selecting appropriate remedies for individual patients. Homeopathy does not tell you what medicine to use in such and such a case, it gives a very precise guideline on how to select the best possible remedy for each case to achieve rapid, smooth and lasting improvement (cure) for each patient, regardless of what the diagnosis may be. Homeopathy is a remedy selection technique aimed at finding an appropriate remedy for each individual patient.

The second feature of homeopathy is the guidance it gives on how to determine the direction in which the patient is evolving. Just the disappearance of a symptom is not sufficient to talk about a homeopathic cure. The improvement has to engage the total patient and establish itself in a well-defined manner often referred to as the Law of Hering. A cure obeying the homeopathic healing concept is a guarantee for smooth improvement and lasting results.

> Note: The Law of Hering says that the patient should improve as if he goes back in time: the latest symptoms to have appeared should disappear first. Sometimes previous symptoms reappear for a short time during the healing process. Ideally they appear in a less dramatic way than the patient experienced them before. Improvement is mostly accompanied by a feel-good situation or an increase in energy, even if the patient still experiences some of his undesired symptoms. It is as if he takes them in his stride more easily.
>
> (The perfect situation is where nothing seems to happen while the patient just gets better and better.) This law is often misinterpreted as the cure by removal of the layers of disease (i.e. peeling of the onion.)

Using this classification, what is generally referred to as Natural Medicine, is experience-based medicine. It will use substances found in nature, based on accumulated knowledge and justify their use through experience and a variety of philosophies about life and illness. These philosophies are the product of life experience and give the various Natural Medicine techniques a more or less appealing character according to one's own understandings and convictions. Different philosophies will produce different results depending on the sensitivity of the practitioner and the patient.

Some of these philosophies are very old like Acupuncture or Ayurvedic medicine and have become very efficient traditions in their own right. The treatment methods these techniques developed over their hundreds of years of history allows them to compete with homeopathy for similar treatment possibilities and effectiveness. Accumulated experience over the years has turned them into efficient systems for individual treatment selection rather than just experience based. To use these techniques with a maximum of success it is necessary to harmonise with the culture that has produced them. As in homeopathy these techniques have often undergone some westernisation to simplify their use. This commonly reduces the long-term benefits that can be expected from these techniques.

There is a second way to divide medical practice into three systems. Hahnemann left his mark on this classification by naming them. The first one he named was homeopathy where like is cured through like; the patient is given a substance that causes a similar suffering to eliminate the condition/symptoms that are present. Desensibilisation in allergic patients and vaccinations also use this principle although their prescription is based on what causes the same. Their effects on the patient are therefore of a different nature than homeopathy.

The second type of prescription is antipathy or enathiopathy; the condition is treated with what causes/does the opposite in the patient. The reaction of the medicine on the patient has the opposite effect compared to the patient's symptoms. This type of medicine includes all treatments that aim at eliminating symptoms by creating an opposite reaction in the patient. Anti-inflammatory therapy, anti-mitotic therapy (cancer drugs), anti-spasmodic in diarrhoea, painkillers, application of cold on bruises, cold water to burns etc, hormonal treatments, are examples of this approach to medicine. Both modern medicine and some herbal treatments use this type of approach. The advantage of this approach is that it often produces quick answers and quick relief. It is a convenient method of medicinal practice but it never cures the patient. It is recognized by many medical practitioners that after using such treatments, the symptoms may come back and often with increased intensity. In other cases the disease will disappear from where it occurred previously to 'travel' to another location in the patient and start a different disease.

The third type is allopathy or heteropathy; there is no relationship between the symptoms caused by the medicine on the patient and the aspect of disease expressed by the patient. A typical example of this type of practice is the use of antibiotics. Surgical interventions are also allopathic in nature. Antibiotics do not use their action on the patient to achieve the effect that is desired from them; the purpose of their use is to eliminate the bacteria that are considered to be the cause of a disease. Antibiotics may have a toxic effect on (some) patients but it is not through this action that they are supposed to achieve their effects until somebody realized that a particular antibiotic is effective when a patient shows certain symptoms. A very experienced physicist explained to me not long ago how he had noticed that Rimfapicine was very effective in eliminating a certain type of rash and itch in people who suffer with liver problems. He now uses this antibiotic when patients complain of such symptoms with the sole purpose of relieving the patient, not to eliminate a specific germ. Experience based medicine in this example offered the possibility of using this particular antibiotic in a 'homeopathic' way instead of its allopathic use.

Another example of this third kind of medicine is the wide variety of treatments that aim at 'eliminating' disease, toxins, suffering. The effect (the 'toxic' reaction of the medicine on the patient) these treatments have on the patient are not related to the symptoms of the patient or the symptoms they can generate in a healthy person; they are supposed to do something for the patient, as if they help him out. The old fashioned technique of bleeding is a classic example but many more treatments exist; they may be aimed at stimulating the liver, immune system, blood flow, etc.

The antipathic techniques are likely to be the less efficient forms of long-term curing; their advantage is that they are convenient to use, rapid in their action but they only bring relief; they help out the patient like a pair of crutches. The crutches don't heal the broken leg but help the patient overcome his temporary incapacity.

Allopathy has an importance in saving lives in very acute circumstances. When a long-term cure of the patient is desired, other techniques will have to follow the first line, antipathic defence or interference with the disease process.

In this puzzle of different techniques we have to make choices. Often these choices are based on personal or other's experiences. To judge what has worked for others or ourselves we have to define what can be considered as efficient. A common cold cured in 4 days with an antibiotic (or a homeopathic remedy) proves nothing. It is even likely that the common cold would have disappeared more quickly without the use of the antibiotic (or homeopathic remedy). To compare the efficiency of an antibiotic with another 'reference' antibiotic (common way of testing the effectiveness of new drugs in conventional medicine) proves nothing. Maybe the condition that was tested would have disappeared more quickly with good hygienic measures (rest, appropriate food and drink, clean air and bedding) faster than by using any antibiotic!

J. Moureau (a French pediatrician) wrote in his book on pragmatism in homeopathy how he discovered that by using homeopathy as a first line prescription, in the cases where the homeopathic prescription did not make any difference, children used to get better quicker than when they were given conventional treatments. He (and that should be the norm!) considers that if the homeopathic prescription does not completely resolve the case of an acute disease in less then 48 hrs, the homeopathic prescription is not responsible for the improvement of the child.

What he also noticed is that when an appropriate antibiotic was given on the second or the third day (to appease anxious parents) after insufficient homeopathic result, the antibiotic was often efficient soon after its first administration. This seemed a more effective way of using antibiotics than starting them from day one

Two explanations may be used for this: the homeopathic remedy that wasn't capable of curing the patient did initiate some reaction that only needed a little extra help from the antibiotic to terminate the healing.

The other explanation may be that antibiotics work better when infection has set in. Infection usually only establishes itself after the first stage of the disease. Bacteria tend to appear after the first initial inflammation phase; bacteria are a normal complication of disease. When antibiotics are given before the infection appears they may influence the future progress of the disease in a harmful way. This may be because they have an influence on the selection of the bacteria that will establish after the beginning of the disease, or can be due to the (unexpected) toxic effect on the patient or by preventing less harmful bacteria from appearing in the patient after the initial inflammation of the starting disease, because of their anti-bacterial effect.

Care is needed with this last reasoning when we talk about chronic reoccurring disease in older patients. It is important to differentiate between real acute diseases and chronic reoccurring diseases in determining treatment strategies.

If a medicine does not bring 'instant' relief in an acute manifestation it cannot be considered efficient; it will be very difficult to distinguish between the action of the medicine and the part of natural healing. 'Successful treatment' after 7 days in an infectious disease can scarcely be labelled successful.

It becomes a little more difficult to decide on efficiency in chronic disease. Efficiency has to be decided by the 'holistic' nature of the improvement and the non-appearance of setbacks where disease reappears or is replaced by other diseases.

Homeopathic dilutions.

In Hahnemann's time, there were no precision instruments to measure and make the high dilutions he wished to use. To overcome this problem, he developed a system of step-by-step diluting using the same amount of the same solvent in each step. This assured reproduction of the dilution level so that information could be recorded precisely and exchanged with others. It is only later that Hahnemann realised that the mixing action (i.e. shaking) between each dilution step to assure homogeneity was important to 'release' the activity of his new medicines.

The system works as follows:

Plants, salts, animal extracts or other substances that dissolve in water are macerated and mixed into a 90% alcohol solution. Substances that cannot be dissolved in water like metals or other minerals are ground into lactose (i.e. milk sugar) using a mortar. These mixtures are called the Mother Tinctures and are the starting points for homeopathically diluted preparations.
(Mother Tinctures are also used in herbal medicine.)

Depending on the type of dilution that is requested, one part of the Mother Tincture is added to 9 or 99 parts of the solvent. This will produce the 1D or 1C solution. Dilution levels are at this point one in ten or one in a hundred.
The solvent is 70% alcohol for water-soluble substances and lactose for substances that cannot be dissolved in water.
It is then important to shake (or grind in a mortar if lactose is used) this mixture thoroughly to assure a homogenous mix and also to assure that the solution is dynamised. Dynamisation refers to the influence of the energetic mixing between diluting steps that assures the 'release' of the homeopathic action of the prepared dilution.
(Hahnemann used this energetic mixing to assure the homogeneity of his preparations. Only later did he discover how important this mixing was to 'release' the activity of his new remedies. Since then this mixing has been known as dynamisation)

In the next step the same process is repeated starting from the 1st dilution level by adding one part of the 1D or 1C dilution to 9 or 99 parts of solvent to prepare a 2D or a 2C dilution. This is then followed again by a good mixing action.

When the 4th dilution is obtained by using lactose as a dilutant, the next step will be to use 70% alcohol to produce the next dilution. This further facilitates the dilution process.

Dilution steps can continue to 30C and even 200C. This means that 30 or 200 one in a hundred dilution steps have been taken.

Two other common diluting techniques are the one in 49,999 parts dilution technique to prepare a high diluted remedy that has received few dynamisations (i.e. vigorous mixing) influence and the Korsakov (K) dilutions.

To prepare a K dilution the solvent is added to the vial that contained the previous dilution. This vial is emptied leaving a few traces of the previous dilution on the walls. The amount of solvent that is added to this emptied vial is approximately 99 parts to 1 part of original dilution left in the vial. The new solution then undergoes the usual shaking action for mixing/dynamisation purpose. Therefore there is no great difference between a Korsakov dilution and a C dilution.

The Korsakov technique has lent itself to mechanical preparation and is therefore now a technique of choice to prepare very high-diluted remedies in modern labs.

These very high-diluted remedies may go up to 1000 and even ten and fifty thousand steps. If they were to be prepared manually this would take a considerable amount of time.

Hahnemann mostly used the one in 99 steps. There were other dilution types developed over time. I haven't mentioned them because they have gone out of fashion or are not frequently used.

Dilutions are often classified as low, medium or high.

The D (one in ten) dilutions are low diluted until they reach the 50D level (i.e. 50 times one in ten dilution). Over this level they will be medium diluted and over 120 steps high diluted.

A 10D dilution compares with a 1C dilution when comparing for the concentration of the diluted substance. The difference between these two dilutions is the amount of dynamisations the solution has undergone. A 10D solution will therefore be more 'energetic' than a 1C solution. This doesn't mean it is more effective from a homeopathic point of view. Its activity on the patient will be more pronounced or visible.

C dilutions are called low dilutions up to 6C and high dilutions from 12C onwards.

LM dilutions (one in a 49,999) are high dilutions that have undergone few dynamisations. The advantage of this kind of dilution is that their effect is generally of a milder character. They are therefore indicated in very sensitive patients (i.e. asthma patients) or when the totality of the patient has greatly improved using a remedy and some extra activity is desired on a local plan using the same remedy. At the same time the use of a LM dilution may be a good way to test the homeopathicity (i.e. good homeopathic activity on the patient) of a remedy for the patient.

Generally speaking, the more the prescription is based on the totality of the patient the higher the dilution may be for a successful prescription. This means that the more one can be assured that a remedy will be homeopathic (i.e. type of activity) the higher the dilution of the remedy may be for the benefit of the patient.

The term generally used by homeopaths for dilutions is potencies. This refers to the fact that a remedy is both diluted and dynamised (i.e. made potent.)

It is often said that the higher a substance is diluted the stronger its effect will be. A stronger homeopathic medicine does not mean a greater efficiency for the patient. By increasing the dilution (or potency) of a remedy we increase the possibility of having a greater impact on the patient (or medicine tester), a greater impact in the sense that its effect will have a profound and long acting influence on the patient. For this impact or influence to be of a healing kind it is essential that the administered remedy is homeopathic to the patient. It is always more important to select the right remedy than to select between a high or medium diluted remedy.

Note: I am sometime horrified to see how in certain leaflets it is proposed to use remedies in 30C or 200C dilution in a repeated way. I remember somebody complaining that when she (on advice from a homeopathic pharmacy) took several doses of Symphytum 200 to help in healing her broken arm, a very uncomfortable pain in her shoulder appeared. This pain was not related to the trauma and she had never experienced it before. When the remedy was stopped the pain disappeared. The pain was the consequence of an 'abuse' of the homeopathic remedy.

In another case a pony with laminitis (painful condition of the feet) was treated with a combination of remedies in a 200C dilution (sent after a telephone conversation with a company that promotes his 'specialised homeopathic remedies for horses') and administered daily. After 15 days the pain in the hooves had disappeared but the pony was anxious, restless, not knowing what to do with itself; it was sad to see how he behaved in his box! When the remedies were stopped he settled down and of course the pain in the hooves came back because the prescription had no curing effect at all on this case. It is very annoying to see such practices of homeopathy where commercial interests win over the interest of the patient.

Low diluted remedies (and most D dilutions) are indicated when a prescription is based on local symptoms only and a less 'homeopathic' action of the remedy is expected. Often, the remedy will be repeated several times over a shorter or longer time span.

The decision of dilution and repetition of a remedy also depends whether one uses homeopathy in acute complaints or chronic complaints.

By using the term potency, it is easier to specify the 'energy' of a preparation. Although a 7C and 70D potency have the same level of dilution, the 70D potency has undergone more mixing steps (dynamisations) and is therefore more potent then the 7C.

When high dilutions are forced upon a patient (i.e. through repetition) without giving the chance/time to react to the remedy, there is a chance that the sensitivity of the patient is altered. The consequence of this may be very positive in the short term; the patient can feel good under the influence of such a remedy. In the long term, cases have a tendency to become more complicated or confused. When the remedy is stopped or the sensitivity of the patient to the remedy changes, it becomes often obvious that the patient hasn't been cured at all. Often the disease has shifted somewhere else or to a deeper more dangerous level.

Too frequent use of homeopathic prepared medicines can have three consequences.

1) The remedy is forced onto the patient and he will develop symptoms belonging to the remedy. This is called a proving or remedy testing because that is the way substances are tested on healthy experimentees before they become homeopathic remedies. The patient reacts to the remedy but its administration brings no cure.

2) In some patients the remedy will after a short period stop the initial benefit it may have produced. It is as if the remedy antidotes itself.

3) Some patients can benefit very well from repeated administration of a remedy. There is no real homeopathic healing action in these cases. The remedy brings the patient into a situation where he can

cope better with his surroundings and therefore feel and appear healthier but it is as if the patient is dependant on the remedy...

I will not go deeper into the subject of the choice of dilution and the repetition of the remedy, because this is a subject were many opinions prevail, and practice differs between homeopaths. The experience of a large proportion of serious homeopaths is that patients make the most appreciable recoveries when the remedy is repeated only very few times. Such practice is more considerate to patients.

Remember that you cannot say that homeopathic remedies can do no harm and at the same time pretend that they are efficient.

Homeopathic dilutions and modern science.

The subject of dilutions is very controversial and is the issue of very animated exchanges with conventional science. Once the dilution of a remedy is past the 9 to 12C (90 –120D) level, according to conventional physical laws, no more original substance can be present in the solution. Much of the criticism towards homeopathy is based on the fact that homeopaths daily use dilutions beyond this level and experience/claim successes with them.

There are several ways to prove that the homeopathic preparation method makes a difference to the obtained solution of a high-diluted substance.

1) The first obvious one is the fact that high-diluted substances are used to test medicines on healthy people. It is the symptoms obtained after the ingestion of high- diluted substances that are used to identify its homeopathic action. This information is then used to select a remedy for the patient.

Anybody who is unwilling to believe this is kindly invited to purchase a preparation of Arsenicum album 30C and take some of this preparation daily for a while. If not convinced about the honest preparation of the purchase, it is possible to dilute the obtained medicine 30 times on in a hundred before starting this personal test.

2) There are several experiments recorded that have been checked on the quality of their scientific standards by a peer group of scientists which clearly show that homeopathic diluted substances can make a difference using correctly performed trials. Even if they are not a proof of efficiency of homeopathic prescription, they prove that homeopathically diluted medicines have an influence on people, animals and even cell cultures. After having accepted the validity of the structure of these experiments using homeopathically diluted remedies, their results have been rejected because no rational explanation was proposed or found to explain these results.

3) Recent efforts by scientists using modern high-tech measuring techniques have shown that the solution obtained using the homeopathic dilution technique has undergone physical changes. Electron microscopes, light emission techniques and spectro-photometers are capable of detecting differences between the solvent and a homeopathic dilution of a substance using the same solvent and this when dilutions went beyond the 'fatal' 12C mark.

Over the last few decades there has been a growing interest from science to experiment with high-diluted substances. This may lead one day to the official recognition that homeopathic medicines have a reason to exist but it is still far off because this scientific work does not have many commercial interests in comparison to the pharmaceutical industry which sponsors and promotes research and marketing of modern medicines.

Much work is done on the theory of water clusters. Due to the physical influence (energetic mixing) of a dissolved substance on the solvent (water) this solvent will be organised in a specific way. When we observe water it appears to be an unorganised mixture of water molecules (and contaminants) mostly influenced by external forces that act on it.

Over the last few years a new line of research has been very interested in the organisation of water molecules around other molecules that are dissolved in it. Under the influence of energetic shaking, the water molecules will organise themselves in various layers, thus forming a sort of negative imprint of the original molecule. When a substance is dissolved using the homeopathic step by step principle, these negative imprints of water molecules will stay present even when the solution is so much diluted that no initial substance is present any more. These imprints (or clusters) are stable in time. When agitated they even have a tendency to reproduce further copies of themselves. This new concept sounds to be a contradiction of our common understanding of the behaviour of water molecules in their liquid state. The presence of these clusters can be detected with a certain type of spectro-photometry; they can be scientifically detected.

There is a commercial lab in the US that produces concentrates of such clusters and commercialises them for use in research and certain applications in the petroleum industry.

Anybody who is open minded enough should be able to find sufficient proof to become convinced about the reality of high-diluted remedies. The next step is then to accept that a different way of approaching medicine, different from conventional and rational ideas has a place in this world and is capable of making a big difference in patient's health by using these diluted medicines.

Note: In a recent article in Homeopathic Links, an international journal on homeopathy, a scientist explained how he examined, with a technique called light emission, the change in the concentration of the contaminants that are always present in very low amounts in 'pure' (distilled) water solutions. When he prepared homeopathic dilutions by using 'pure' water and a salt, the concentrations of these very small amounts of contaminants that were present in the 'pure' water used as the solvent, changed significantly even when dilution continued beyond the level at which the salt that was added in the beginning could not be detected in the obtained solution anymore (dilution past the critical number). Changes were different when different salts were diluted.

He suggested that when a homeopathic preparation was administered to a living organism, the organism would 'recognise' a typical change in the composition of the solvent caused by the originally diluted substance. The typical change in the contaminants is accompanied by the absence of the substance that had caused this change. This 'contradiction' may trigger off a reaction from the organism that expects to undergo a poisoning from the original substance at first glance from the information carried by the solvent but does not encounter the poisonous agent it expects to find.

This summary of a long article is an example of how modern science (physics) is slowly progressing towards the possibility of recognition of homeopathically prepared remedies.

What homeopathic remedies are made from and the difference of homeopathy to herbal medicine.

A common confusion exists between herbal medicine and homeopathy. This is mainly because many homeopathic remedies are prepared from plants. That is where the comparison ends.

As explained in previous chapters, the above named medicinal techniques are based on different prescription modes. The reason why one plant is used in homeopathy differs from the reason why the same plant is used in herbal medicine.

Sometimes it is difficult to draw the line between the two techniques because herbs are commonly used homeopathically prepared but based on their herb-medicine indications. This is herbal medicine making use of the homeopathic preparation technique. Also, homeopathy makes use of herbal knowledge about plants to develop a homeopathic vision on their possible use. Herbal information on plants may be used in the homeopathic remedy selection process.

In the interest of patients it is important that both techniques are regarded as very different.

When Hahnemann started to test various substances when he was discovering homeopathy, he mainly used substances that were already in use as medicines because he wanted to find the proper indications of these medicines through his new scientific testing method. He started with China, then Belladonna then followed Arsenicum album, Veratrum album, Mercurius, etc.: all medicines used in his time. Over the years a variety of other substances have been used to detect their homeopathic activity. Not only flowers, plants and trees but also many minerals, metals, toxins, venoms and other human and animal derived products have been put to the test and are commonly used as homeopathic remedies.

The reasons for the substance selection for homeopathic testing are as various as the people that have orchestrated these tests. Nowadays, for instance, substances like plastic, Coca Cola, plutonium nitricum, eagle blood, human milk, diamond, marble, hydrogenium and many others have joined the ranks of homeopathic tested remedies. Any substance can become a homeopathic remedy under the condition that a correctly practised proving (i.e. test) has been conducted that produced significant symptoms.

Like cures like.

The principle that like can cure like has been present in many medical traditions. Examples are found in historic references of Indian, Arabian and European (Greek) origins. In old medical treatises originating in these cultures, treatments are often discussed using both the 'like cures like' principle and the 'opposing' principle leaving the choice to the practitioner. The third type of treatment refers to hygiene in the large sense of the word. Living conditions, eating habits, exercise of body and mind and even 'counselling' fall into this third method.

In our modern world where logic prevails, it seems obvious that the normal way of treating disease is by eliminating its symptoms or supposed causes. 'Like cures like' gives the impression that we will make disease worse by adding 'extra disease' to the patient.

One example that shows how 'like cures like' defies logic is the following: Logic says that in case of burning, the skin should be held under cold water to cool down, stop the burning process and trigger an anti-inflammatory process through cold application.

If we think a little further using our knowledge of blood circulation, anatomy and physics, it is obvious that any heat present in the burned skin will be eliminated within less then a second due to the large amounts of blood that flows in the small vessels just under the skin (this is one of the reasons why some people manage to run over hot coals). There is no need to use cold water to bring down the temperature and stop the heat effect. By the time we reach the tap, the heat has already disappeared and we only feel the burning of the heat. The cold water running on the burn stops the burning feeling.

The only satisfying reason to use cold water is to try and stop a (too severe) inflammation reaction that may sometimes aggravate the original lesions by using the 'freezing' effect of cold. This is an example of treating by using the anti or opposing principle.

'Like cures like' advises bringing the burned skin again close to (not against!) a heat source until the heat becomes uncomfortable again (often 5 to 20 seconds) and then remove the burned body part to let it settle without interfering.

I tried this second option several times when my occupations in the kitchen caused me to burn a finger or my hand and I can assure you that the pain in the burned skin disappears very quickly (less than one hour), that there are no after pains and that the burn lesion heals quickly and uneventfully without the need of water, ointments or other applications. I used this system for both second and third degree burns and found it very satisfying, much more than the conventional reflex of cooling down. This is something everybody can test. When we cool down burns under cold water we take away the pain very quickly only for it to reappear later and linger on for quite a while.

Be careful with serious burns!!!

A less dramatic example is the application of cold water to hands or feet that have been cooled down painfully in cold weather. After that, they should be left to warm up slowly. The advantage of doing this is that there will be much less uncomfortable tingling in the hands or feet when they warm up.

I am sure that many have seen old films where a patient with high fever is wrapped into blankets and brought close to a warm fire 'to sweat out the disease'. Reasoning tells us to cool down somebody with a high fever; this is not proven at all and in most occasions does not benefit the patient at all.

In farming traditions people used to have a small strong alcoholic drink when they were hot from labouring in the summer sun. Only after having cooled in the shade for a while, would they drink the amounts of water they needed. This eliminates the chance of vertigo or colic from drinking cold water.

There are many more examples of the 'like cures like' principle that can be found in popular habits and wisdom.

What can be treated with homeopathy?

The answer to this question is that the possibilities are unlimited. It is obvious that a wound needs stitching and a broken leg or dislocated joint needs mending. Most other diseases or symptoms, whether they are mental illnesses, coughs, abscesses, tumours or immune diseases, are all the result of some 'faulty' or excessive or inactive body function. As long as the damage that has occurred during the disease process is not beyond repair (a limit difficult to determine) there is always a possibility of finding a homeopathic remedy that will make a big difference in the outcome or even achieve a spectacular cure. Disease is the result of an action of the body/mind and will express itself through physical and/or psychological symptoms. Given the appropriate information/help in the form of a homeopathic remedy, the body/mind will be able to restore what has gone wrong and the disease symptoms will disappear. The limit of homeopathic efficiency is determined by the possibility of finding as perfect as possible a remedy for the individual patient and the amount of wear and tear the patient has already suffered. Wear and tear does not reflect the severity of the lesions; it is the ability of a patient to recover reflected by the amount of life energy that is left in them.

It is obvious that disturbing circumstances caused by severe unhygienic influences will severely diminish the possibility for improvement with homeopathic remedies if they are not attended to. The most important bad hygienic influences are these that are forced upon the patient: the one on which he has no influence (weather, housing, mistreatment by third parties). If they cannot be changed, it is often difficult to obtain spectacular results with homeopathic prescription although it may be possible to offer some relief to the patient or give the patient the strength to extract himself from such a negative influence.

The patient's own bad hygienic habits may often be corrected by a good homeopathic prescription (smoking, drinking). The bad habit of a patient can be classified as one of his symptoms and be the result of his personal 'sensitivity' that can be changed/improved by an efficient homeopathic prescription.

In some cases the result of the disease process becomes a threat to the patient, as in cancers or severe heart disease. Although a perfect homeopathic treatment may be the ideal solution, conventional intervention may be life and time saving. Efficient and tried conventional treatments should not be discarded. In the meantime it is possible to give homeopathy the chance and the time to improve obtained results and ensure that they last. Decisions in these cases have to be made individually. There is no harm in trying to benefit from various techniques that are on offer as long as the respect of the patient and not the principles of the physician are put to the forefront.

The question is not so much whether homeopathy is indicated but whether the client/patient is motivated to put in the effort and, sometimes the patience, needed to obtain an efficient homeopathic prescription that will solve the problem or improve the results after conventional (medical or surgical) intervention.

In diseases where there is a lack of production of hormones or other substances, the appropriate homeopathic prescription can only achieve results if enough viable tissue is still present to regenerate normal production. Patients with diabetes will need insulin. A good homeopathic prescription may reduce the dose of insulin or facilitate the stabilisation of the patient. Homeopathy will only cure the patient from diabetes if this is 'technically' possible; where the body is capable of starting to produce its own insulin again.

In chronic ailments, like skin problems, it is sometimes necessary to accept that local symptoms may linger for a while before they disappear while inside the patient a silent revolution is taking place that eliminates one by one all the symptoms and diseases. This should happen in the reverse order to which they have appeared. (Law of Hering)

Instead of asking whether homeopathy is indicated for a given problem, one should question whether there is a need and desire to use homeopathy and whether one is motivated to put in the required effort.

No ailment, no health problem, no behaviour problem or fear is too serious not to be able to benefit from a good homeopathic prescription. Only, the more serious the problem, the more precise the prescription needs to be.

Success often depends on the joint efforts of patient/client and practitioner. Because Classical homeopathy caters for each individual patient it offers a greater chance of finding the most appropriate remedy for each case than any other derived prescription technique that uses homeopathic remedies.

Homeopathy and conventional diagnosis.

I have already repeated several times that the conventional diagnosis is not a good starting point for the selection of a homeopathic remedy in a case.

This doesn't mean that making a diagnosis is of no use. There are several reasons why the diagnosis has its importance in medicine.

In conventional medicine, the principal reason is that the diagnosis will decide the treatment. This principle has given the diagnosis a central place in medicine. Because of this central place in official medicine, diagnosis has acquired a central place in our society. The functioning of our society with regulations, law, insurance, uses diagnosis of disease in its working mechanism. A diagnosis and the knowledge about what we can expect from the diagnosis helps us to understand what the odds are in each case. In many cases it makes us sceptical towards the possible positive outcome when conventionally it is considered that there is no cure. Judging the possibilities for cure only through conventional filters is reducing the chances for the patient.

The desire to know the cause of disease is as old as mankind. Throughout the history of medicine there are many examples of the different efforts made by man to explain and 'justify' disease.

Finding this cause is straightforward when the 'disease' is the consequence of an identifiable injury. Injury is like an attack and can take the form of physical injury but also of a poisoning, bad habits, obvious psychological injury, climatic 'attacks', epidemics, etc.

Things become unclear when one morning we wake up not feeling well or when patients develop chronic disease. No obvious cause seems to explain why the disease started. It is often the case that patients dwell for a while between various examinations or, in some cases, forever without receiving a satisfactory answer to their demand to find out what is wrong with them or what caused the onset of the disease or their suffering.

Throughout history explanations for such 'disease' have been determined by the prevailing cultural ideas. Over the last two hundred years, with the improvements in modern medicine, the causes of 'unexplainable' diseases have become more and more 'objective'. Objective means: shown through image, post mortem, blood result, analysis of urine, proof of the presence of bacteria, auscultation. The patient has a streptococcus bacterium, has a lung abscess, has a bladder inflammation or has a tumour. This gives a justification of his ill-being; the patient is given a right to be ill because it is known why he is not well; an objective measurement of his disease can be made.

At first the diagnosis or explanation of the disease was there to be a safeguard for efficient treatment. Over the last hundred years, there has arisen a demand from health service consumers for a diagnosis or explanation of their disease and this is now a 'right' they have acquired. The results from examinations made become very important. Things have gone so far that many patients talk about 'their' blood results, 'their' scan, 'their' X-ray results and how good or bad their results are doing.

Diagnosis satisfies our natural desire to know or understand what is happening. With the advance of science, statistics and recording, the medical world has acquired a huge amount of information on the link between diagnosis and prognosis. Therefore by making a diagnosis we not only receive a sense of understanding but equally an idea as to what generally can be expected from the evolution of a disease or condition. This is very satisfying and gives the feeling of being in control.

Diagnosis has become a right and is expected by the health consumer. It gives the feeling that the health practitioner, who makes the diagnosis, knows what he is doing. Naming a disease gives us the feeling that the disease is real; we feel more comfortable about it because it allows us to discuss the disease with friends or surf the Net for more information. After having shared our diagnosis with others we suddenly feel less lonely. Exchange with others has an effect of counselling which is in itself a medical technique that can bring some improvement. Diagnosis has become so important that many patients are satisfied with medicine as soon as they receive 'their' diagnosis. Whether there is a solution for their problem or not seems to matter less. When conventional medicine tells them there is no solution, many seem to accept this as their fate. How often do we hear a patient saying: "The doctor found what I have. There is no treatment" and this same patient being very satisfied with the doctor's service.

By reducing the patient to the result of an examination, we forget the individual behind the suffering. Several patients with the same X-ray or blood results can suffer very differently. Patients with 'normal' results can suffer while others with 'abnormal' results can feel very well.

On many occasions the 'diagnosis' or objective finding is the (end) result of a disease/illness/suffering that has been present for a while. The patient has been feeling unwell/complaining for a while and after many attempts to make a diagnosis finally something is found. This may be because enough time has elapsed since the beginning of the complaint for the objectivable part (i.e. that which can be proven to be abnormal in the patient using a physical examination, through imaging, lab results or other technique) of the disease to become 'findable' (i.e. able to be found or proven by a modern examination.)

The objectivisation of disease is carried out by using modern science. Because of the value/importance that is given to modern science, modern diagnosis is perceived to be of high value. Science has been extremely efficient in reducing nature around and inside us to measurable and calculable values that can be used successfully to interfere with these natural phenomena. What science has never been able to cater for are the small differences between patients that make them individuals.

In homeopathic medicine, the diagnosis has an importance in the communication with the client/patient. It is important to make decisions on the strategy of prescription. The diagnosis will also help in selecting the 'homeopathic' symptoms by determining what are the specific symptoms in the individual case and what are the common symptoms in the case.

Homeopathy makes its own type of diagnosis.

The first type of diagnosis is the selection of the appropriate remedy for the case. The second type of diagnosis is the holistic view on the severity of the disease and the evolution of the case after prescription. This will decide whether the evolution of the patient after prescription is favourable. It is not uncommon that according to conventional terms the patient has improved after the use of homeopathic remedies but that from a homeopathic point of view the evolution of the patient has not been favourable in the long term.

Conventionally it is often not possible to explain the connection between different diseases that affect the patient. If no scientific or reasoned link has been established between different features in a patient it is considered that there is no link. Modern medicine treats us like a machine that is the sum of its body parts. We are more than the sum of our body parts; there is something that holds them together and influences them that we cannot measure.

The homeopathic holistic approach does not try to explain the connection between different diseases but considers that all that happens in the patient is an expression of the patient's 'chronic' disease (i.e. inner working mechanism).

When one disease is later 'replaced' by another disease that evolves in a more important part of the body/mind, this is considered as an aggravation in homeopathic medicine. A classical homeopath will conclude that his previous prescription may have satisfied the patient but has not improved the patient in the long run. He knows he has to find a better remedy for the patient.

The purpose of classical homeopathic prescription goes further than eliminating the patient's complaint for which he consulted. Practitioners try to improve the patient is such a way that they not only eliminate their suffering but find themselves in a much better harmony with their environment and peace within.

The World Health Organisation defines health as the well-being of an individual in his body, mind and surroundings. Health is not defined as a sum of objective measurements and images that are within what is considered to be normal; it is defined by the well-being, good feeling, balanced living of an individual in his surroundings. Both the surroundings (hygiene) and the individual play a role. The need for individualisation can be understood by the common observation that for different people, different situations are considered to be comfortable.

There are even people and animals that are healthy with 'abnormal' blood results. There is a danger that in some cases modern medicine declares them 'unhealthy', or makes them feel unhealthy, by telling them that they are at risk of such and such a disease.

Things may become worse by screening for 'genetic' factors that indicate a certain risk of disease. 'Patients' may be told at a 'young' age what future problems they will encounter ... but without accompanying adequate solutions for help. The technical development of modern medicine not only brings improved medicine but also puts many new strains on moral issues.

Homeopathy and concepts of disease.

It is common to hear about psora, sycosis and syphilis when reading on the subject of homeopathy. The following will help you understand what place the concept of psora and the other chronic diseases takes in homeopathic medicine.

When Hahnemann had already discovered the particularities of homeopathic prescription and written his first edition of the Organon explaining them, he was still learning how to apply these particularities in daily practice.

This seems to be a contradiction: knowing how homeopathy should be practised and at the same time finding it difficult to apply this in daily practice but this is the brilliant contribution of Hahnemann to medicine; he saw what was important to make homeopathic remedies work before he mastered the technique. This is a common feature of homeopathic medicine. The homeopathic principles are not very complicated to understand. The application of these principles to practise good homeopathic prescription demands a great effort. The cause of this is the very nature of homeopathy that aims at treating the individual rather than the disease. By concentrating on treating the individual, the variability in prescription possibilities becomes endless because every individual may express his 'ill-being' in a different way and therefore need a different prescription.

During his pursuit to improve his prescriptions, he observed how patients had a tendency to reproduce certain of their symptoms over and over again. When they disappeared, patients often produced different and sometimes worse symptoms. After many years of observing his patients, he determined patterns in the ways chronic illness evolves. He then proposed a classification of these chronic diseases into three forms.

He called them psora, sycosis and luesis due to their resemblance with three of the more common diseases of his time:

- Scabies or mange, a skin disease caused by tiny parasites that was the most common cause of itching in his time.

- Gonorrhea, a sexually transmitted disease, causing chronic discharges and the formation of polyps on and around the sexual organs (related to the presence of a gonococcus bacteria).

- And syphilis, another sexually transmitted disease, causing inflammations, ulcers and disease of the nerves (related to the presence of a treponema bacteria).

These three different diseases are also called 'miasmas'. A miasma can be seen as a precursor to what we now call infectious agents. A patient could be infected by one or two or even three miasmas which were the inner causes for the patient's chronic diseases and/or symptoms. These 'infections' could be acquired through birth (hereditary) or could be acquired during life, usually as a consequence of 'bad' habits or lack of hygiene. (The case of gonorrhea and syphilis) Each particular disease would cause certain types of symptoms to appear; they are decided on by the dynamics of the evolution of the patient.

This original concept of classification of chronic recurring and changing symptoms, created by Hahnemann, has since then been used, adapted and discussed by many homeopaths through homeopathic history and up to now.

Hahnemann 'discovered' them because he was looking for ways to improve the prescription of his new medicines in the face of the difficulties he encountered in treating chronic disease successfully. When he published his findings, they were supposed to help the homeopathy in orientating his prescriptions but maybe they also served as an explanation for the lack of satisfying success.

The subject of the study of these chronic diseases is vast and has filled many books and discussions

In summary, different explanations have led to a variety of different models that are supposed to help improving or facilitating homeopathic prescription. Following are a few examples of how the models of chronic disease are used in a variety of ways to help in the selection of remedies:

- Chronic disease models have been (and still are) used to classify remedies according to their activity on symptoms that are associated with one of these chronic diseases. This facilitates the selection of remedies after having determined which chronic disease(s) is present in the patient. An appropriate remedy can then be selected out of a smaller group

- By determining the 'chronic disease' of a patient, this is supposed to help in deciding which symptoms are supposed to have an increased value to find the appropriate remedy.

- The notion of chronic disease is also applied to the different aspects the picture of a homeopathic remedy can take. Three patients may benefit from the same homeopathic remedy while their 'personal disease picture' can be very different. In a simplified way we can illustrate this like the following:
* A psoric condition will cause the expression of behaviour and disease to be related with the surroundings in a dynamic way,
* A sycotic condition will create an image of a patient locked in himself with slow continuous disease that has a tendency to 'build'.
* A syphilitic condition has a more 'destructive' appearance (towards others or themselves)
If the remedy's disease picture is related to security, this can be expressed depending on the chronic disease expression by: friendliness to other people in search for protection (psora), somebody who isolates himself (sycosis) or somebody who is very manipulative in his relations (syphilis). This allows the homeopath to use the same remedy in what appears to be very

different cases. Once it has been established/suspected what drives the patient towards certain reactions, the same remedy can be given based on the 'underlying theme' even if at first the cases looked very dissimilar.

- There is a renowned Indian homeopath (R. Sankaran) who has enlarged the number of chronic diseases that can be recognised in patients from three to twelve. He also has started to classify remedies in groups that have a common 'sensitivity'. Within each group, remedies are classified according to which one of the 12 chronic diseases they belong (i.e. way of reacting). When the practitioner can determine the sensitivity of the patient, this will indicate a particular group of remedies. According to the type of chronic disease the patient expresses, one of the remedies in the group will be indicated.

For some, the study of chronic diseases is a guidance that helps them in their daily practice. I will not treat this subject in depth. That would take hundreds of pages and has more philosophical and historical importance. Throughout the history of homeopathy and depending who talks about them, definitions of chronic diseases and importance attached to them tend to vary from homeopath to homeopath and school to school. It does not have its place in a presentation about homeopathic medicine because it may take the attention away from what is essential to know about homeopathy.

It is quite possible to practise very good homeopathy without using such concepts. Many do this.

One of the reasons why Hahnemann found his success-rate too low was because of his desire for excellence. Another reason is that he had not enough experience with the new medicines AND the technique he just discovered. Progress has been made since then and is still going on at a fast pace. There are also more remedies experimented on than during Hahnemann's time, allowing for more choices for different patients. This has improved results of homeopathic prescription in chronic disease but has not always diminished the popularity of these concepts.

We all like to have a framework in which we can situate both our own and other's diseases. The way homeopathy looks at disease and cure has created substance for the development of these disease concepts. They are often very elegant and inspiring as an alternative to more modern and rigid disease explanations.

Like with so many things, the truth is where it works for you. The discussion around chronic disease and the use of chronic disease concepts are a framework within which homeopathy can be practised. But it is important not to forget that homeopathy is about finding and determining the patient's homeopathic symptoms followed by the selection of the appropriate remedy that is indicated by these symptoms to achieve rapid and smooth healing in the patient. The use of chronic disease concepts may help in the selection of the appropriate remedy but is best not to be seen as obligatory for good prescription.

Psora is nowadays mostly associated with the central delusion or sensitivity of the patient that governs most of his psychological and physical reactions. Psora is therefore seen as the inner cause of disease in the patient due to his interaction with his surroundings. In an ideal situation the homeopath will try to find the remedy that will act on this central 'malfunctioning' in order to re-establish a good relation between the patient and his 'surroundings' which will lead to a return to good health. Such a remedy is sometimes called a constitutional remedy.

Homeopathy is often best practised in silence, through observation and listening. Too much talking and explaining can easily drown the essence.

How homeopathy works?

"What does this remedy do?" is a question that is frequently asked when after a long (or short) consultation I tell the client what remedy their pet is going to receive.

From our experience with conventional medicine we are so used to have a 'scientific' explanation for each medicine we take or administer that we expect to receive a similar answer from homeopathy. Modern medicines kill bacteria, stop inflammation, ease pain, relax arteries, stimulate or relax muscle cells, kill cancer cells, interfere with nerve cell receptors, replace or suppress hormones, etc. Such explanations are often well documented and illustrate the major activity of the drugs we use. Such explanations justify the use of a medicine for a specific condition and therefore provide a sense of security and efficacy.

In alternative medicine where scientific explanations are less documented, explanations take on the form of: stimulates the immune system, enhances blood supply, relaxes the mind, treats the soul, soothes the skin, dilutes bile, protects the joints, etc. Where some proof of activity has been gathered herbal medicines are often also classified as antibacterial, anti-inflammatory or stimulating repair. Again these are explanations that give us a sense of purpose for each treatment, herb or mixture that we buy or are prescribed.

The same effort is made for homeopathic prepared substances but explanations are usually less specific: remedies are offered for sale as stimulating the immune system, against diarrhoea, against arthritis, for skin affections, etc. I have explained several times that this approach satisfies a certain demand from the health consumer but that is not very homeopathic and diminishes the long-term chances for the patient.

Saying that a remedy is indicated for a specific disease does not explain how homeopathy works. Explaining the activity of a homeopathic remedy using modern 'scientific' rationale is not possible because there is not yet any generally accepted science that allows for it. There is not enough scientific knowledge that allows us to explain how a high-diluted substance exerts its influence to trigger a healing action. The desire and pressure to use modern science for the explanation of the activity of homeopathic medicines is very high. There are many articles and studies that use quantum mechanic principles, electromagnetic principles and the earlier mentioned water-cluster theories in an effort to deliver some scientific basis to satisfy such demands. The new horizons that are opened through these efforts are very exciting and promising but for the moment offer no satisfactory or generally accepted ideas for the explanation of the activity of homeopathic remedies.

To explain the workings of homeopathy and the value of classical prescription we have to resort to illustrative explanations that help us in understanding how a remedy given only once can make such big changes in the patient.

A very interesting illustration can be found in a book written by R. Sankaran (The Spirit of Homeopathy). He describes how disease can be compared with a mafia organisation. I am going to use this idea and expand it further to gradually build a picture that places the areas in which homeopathic remedies carry out their activity.

In his mafia model, Rajan Sankaran describes how our body is like a country with all the necessary functions for its working. There is a rule of law (genetic code) and police (defense mechanisms) to keep everything in control. When disease creeps in this is like a mafia organisation that infiltrates the country. The presence of the organisation is seen through the presence of dealers on the corners of the street, regular newspaper reports of killings in backyards, money that disappears in the books of big enterprise. These are the tell-tale signs that there is a crime infiltration in the country but nobody can actually see the organisation behind it.

Something similar happens in our body; we all suffer from recurrent symptoms that plague us every so often. In other instances the one or the other body function goes down without obvious reasons. These are the tell signs that there is a 'chronic disease' that operates inside our body like a force or plan that nobody can see. Much work done since C. G. Jung on archetypes, dreams and the relation between mental and physical disease refers to the presence of this underlying mechanism that governs our reactions. This mechanism can be compared with a mafia organisation for the purpose of illustrating how different visible diseases and symptoms all have a relation to each other within the patient and how this complex structure can be tackled in different ways in a more or less efficient way.

It would not be a good idea to say that the each individual's chronic underlying disease is just a mafia organisation and therefore something bad to get rid of as soon as posible; we will find out further that it has also a preserving function.

When the police try to tackle the mafia in the country they can do so by eliminating the dealers on the corners of the street, finding the killers or arresting the fraudulent accountant. These are only the footmen of the mafia organisation and they can be quickly replaced by new recruits. Through such action, the mafia only receives minor blows that it counts as normal collateral damage. Such actions don't stop it continuing to infiltrate the country and create more and more destabilisation and damage.

It is the same for our body; when we deal with symptoms left, right and centre we feel better and are pleased with the temporary victory. Soon 'new recruits' appear and we suffer again. Because we didn't touch the deeper seated disease it can even evolve further and create more damage; it can decide to tackle a more vital part of our body or turn a 'neighborhood' into chaos (tumour, cancer, mental disease).

If the police really want to stop the mafia they have to root out its central command. Observing the petty crime, the pathways of money laundering and unusual behaviour of certain groups will lead them to more higher command levels. When these are taken out much more damage is done to the criminal organisation. It will find it more difficult to re-establish again. The country regains (some of) its healthy functioning and will display a much more buoyant economy.

The purpose of classical homeopathic prescription is very similar; it aims at touching the very inner mechanics and dynamics of the invisible 'chronic disease' that allows various ailments and dysfunctioning to appear at the surface that trouble the patient.

When homeopathic remedies are given to treat a local problem like a disturbed intestine or damaged joint, they most of the time only interfere with this local problem and rarely (only through luck and not through technique) treat the problem at a deeper level. The internal disease of the patient will continue to evolve and new problems (often worse) will sooner or later appear.

The more the remedy is adapted to the patient the more its underlying 'chronic disease' will be stopped in its continuous undermining activity; serious problems can be cured and prevented. When the 'central command' of the disease is touched, most or all the visible signs of the chronic disease will disappear. All the patient's energy can be directed again towards repair and healthy living.

To achieve such a result a remedy needs to be very homeopathic to the patient. The mafia organisation within the patient that behaves like a chronic disease can be illustrated like a wrong/abnormal functioning of the economy. The normal economy is what makes our body/mind function efficiently within our environment. Every individual has its own character, its own ways of reacting to and interacting with the surroundings. When these reactions are efficient, the results are efficient and there is no need for serious disease. Disease should be seen as a way to reduce the damage caused by errors in the general economy of an individual and aggressions from the outside world. Efficient disease activity will target less important structures (mild fever, upper respiratory tract, mouth, intestines, skin) with ailments that cause only temporary inconvenience and soon restore themselves without much need for help. From this viewpoint disease is an efficient defense mechanism that assures the continuity of an individual in the often-hostile environment we live. If we didn't have disease to concentrate all sorts of mishaps into confined areas, the whole economy of our system would go down each time something went wrong or we were confronted with a somewhat stronger attack than usual. A healthy person will have healthy disease reactions. This explains why defense mechanism and disease are the same: The one is the result of inefficient or inept defence reactions the other the result of efficient defence work.

Nobody is perfect; nobody interacts perfectly with his or her surroundings. The way in which our system targets certain functions to suffer the consequences of malfunctioning or interfering external influences is dependant on our particular way of reacting. Serious disease steps in when the individual's reactions become less efficient; when they lose their ability to heal through normal, natural healing or when more important body functions are targeted by the internal disease reaction and life is endangered.

In both the healthy and less healthy disease processes, there are many common reactions we can recognise when we observe different patients but each individual will have a particular combination of reactions or some detail that makes him different from all others.

This particular way of reacting to our own dysfunctions and external influences makes us all individual patients and can be called the dynamics of the individual chronic disease of each patient that determines the symptoms observed by the patient and external observers. They are the characteristics of the patient.

The remedy that is homeopathic to the patient will act on the dynamics of the chronic disease. The remedy is a signal, a trigger that influences the chronic disease of the patient in such a way that it becomes more efficient. An efficient chronic disease can then become an efficient defense mechanism that the patient uses to stay in harmony with his surroundings; that defends the patient efficiently against outside influences and attacks and against the patient's own inefficiencies. Such a remedy acts like a little computer program that helps the inner workings in becoming more efficient.

This illustrates what were these 'new properties' that Hahnemann discovered in his new highly diluted medicines to which I referred in the chapter on the testing of medicine. Instead of causing a poisoning effect on the patient, when diluted according to the homeopathic principles, medicines could become active on the very personal nature of the patient.

Another consequence of this is that when the patient gets in trouble again after having benefited for a long period from such a homeopathic remedy, they often can benefit again from the same remedy to return to 'better efficacy'. This increased efficacy allows them to solve their health problems whether they are physical or psychological.

As explained earlier, there is no real frontier between physical and mental problems; they both belong to the patient and are part of the characteristics that call for the particular remedy: in characteristic is included the word character that refers clearly to the mental part of the patient.

When earlier we discovered how symptoms could be erased like very small replaceable parts of crime activity, larger chunks of disease can also be removed. A mafia organisation relies on different sections each responsible for one aspect of its business. When the police take out one of the sections it will give a serious blow to the organisation and solve a problem in one sector of the country's economy. The core of the mafia still exists and will either rebuild the lost sector, increase its activity in another sector or develop a new business.

What happens in the patient is something very similar, part of the chronic disease responsible for an important illness or suffering can be taken out successfully without restoring the evolution of the underlying chronic disease. This can be done both with homeopathy or other medical techniques. These partial deep cures are much more efficient for the patient then the elimination of a few disturbing symptoms. A typical example in conventional medicine is corrective hip surgery or the surgical removing of cancers and tumours

.

Building on this illustration, the patient's holistic disease scenario may be subdivided into a combination of several smaller diseases operating at the same time. The dynamics of these 'sub'-diseases are often less individual. These sub-diseases can be found and recognised in several patients. A homeopathic remedy that is homeopathic for such a sub-disease will be homeopathic in several patients where a similar sub-disease is flourishing. This means that it will act on the dynamics of a part of the patient's holistic defense reaction. That is why, with a relatively small amount of remedies (200-400), a homeopath can benefit many patients with his prescriptions.

Also the same remedy will be able to act on a series of different disease dynamics scenarios and therefore increase again the possibilities for the homeopath.

Classical homeopathy does not act on disease; it acts on the patient. The remedy that is given to the patient and is able to touch the inner sensitivity of the patient in an efficient way will cause the patient to become more efficient in his defense actions and reactions. As a result symptoms disappear and normal healing become possible again.

If a prescription is less homeopathic or when herbal medicine (or Bach flowers, essential oils, etc.,) are used they act like an encouragement of the normal defense reactions but do not have the deep restoring effect. Their efficiency can be very appreciable but only occasionally (when they happen to be homeopathic to the patient) bring the impressive turnarounds that classical prescription can achieve.

The way in which a remedy acts on the individual can be illustrated in two ways. Both seem contrary but are in fact one.

The appropriate remedy will 'inform' the patient about the 'mafia' activity within their functioning and pushes this activity away. It does this by informing the 'police' activity within the patient and at the same time by imitating the disease. By imitating the disease, the remedy causes an 'artificial' disease that resembles very much (like cures like) a part or totality of the mafia organisation. This artificial disease comes into competition with the 'mafia' activity within the patient (i.e. natural disease which is the disease present in the patient) and therefore reduces its power. This weakens the patient's disease; it is wiped away by the artificial disease caused by the remedy because it engages in the same operations (like competing mafia organisations). This artificial disease is a 'poisoning'. Because the remedy is not repeated (classical homeopathy) the 'poisoning' disappears, leaving behind a weakened natural disease that then can be more efficiently combated or controlled by the normal defense/balance mechanisms within the patient. This illustrates the 'like cures like' activity of the remedy.

By giving a homeopathic remedy to the patient (without too much repetition), they will also 'learn' from the information this remedy brings.

This works in a similar way to when somebody reads a revealing book, hears a revealing speech or has a revealing experience that changes their life. Not the sort of speech or book we like to hear or read over and over again because we like it. It is rather like the sort, that after having heard it or read it once, we rarely have to go back to it for it to have a profound impact on us.

The book we want to read every week to feel better is like the remedy we have to take in regularly to benefit from it. The book we only need to read once can be compared to this really very homeopathic remedy that suited our individuality.

Because of the profound activities they can have on our system (individual being), out of consideration to the patient, is important not to prescribe a remedy on insufficient grounds and certainly manipulate high diluted remedies with caution.

What should be retained from the above journey into a non-conventional vision on disease is that homeopathy is a very lively occupation; nothing is static, nothing is established. The practitioner has endless possibilities to improve the patient. It also explains where the concept of healing by layer and healing on different levels comes from. At the same time it should explain why it is best to guard against trying to apply this concept of healing by layer. It is very presumptuous to affirm that it is possible to recognise the layers that need to be cured in a patient before deciding on a treatment strategy although it is possible and important to recognise after prescription what the path was that the patient took as a result of the remedy and what 'layers' have been touched. It is often obvious that these layers have both horizontal and vertical lines making the cure by layers more of a puzzle than an onion aspect, with each piece of the puzzle often containing different levels of 'activity'. The homeopathic technique gives the homeopath the tools to select a remedy without the need to divide the patient in layers.

The discussion on healing levels belongs to philosophy and education and our understanding that helps us in our perception of health and disease. This in itself can have a healing action and has therefore its own interest. The healing action through philosophical discussions on disease is like the counselling effect psychotherapy can exert on the patient. As said earlier, this form of medicine can be classified as medicine practised through 'hygienic' measures, which can be highly effective.

Another observation is that 'chronic disease' and 'defense mechanism' are terms that can be used for the same concept. This should make us conclude that when possible, respecting disease is always better then eliminating it. Homeopathy is a guiding medicine to help the patient change his underlying, invisible chronic disease into an efficient defense mechanism. The observation that it is important to respect disease is a guidance and should never been taken as a dogma; in some cases the disease is so dangerous that it can destroy the patient. At the same time this observation explains how even in very severe cases that are often considered as incurable, it is always possible to intervene successfully if enough chance is given to both patient and practitioner.

Conclusion.

Homeopathy is distinguished from conventional medicine by accepting the variability that exists between patients. The homeopathic principles of medicine selecting cater for this variety by explaining how to find the best possible medicine for every individual patient and for every individual disease. Opposed to this is modern science which puts great effort into understanding and measuring natural processes and consequently classifying them. By doing this it always reduces reality to abstract rules. The strength of homeopathic prescription is a consequence of its ability to adapt to every patient. The common tendency to introduce modern scientific concepts into homeopathy in an effort to improve its image has always, and will always, result in a diminishing of its adaptability to cater for the individual patient. Therefore, diagnosis orientated homeopathic prescription reduces the possibilities for the patient.

That is why it is worthwhile having an in-depth understanding of the concept of homeopathy. Also, when prescriptions are really tailor-made for the patient, homeopathic prescription does not eliminate symptoms (or diseases). It gives the patient the means to redirect their illness operations in such a way that many or most symptoms (or diseases) become unnecessary and therefore will disappear due to increased efficiency in the patient's operation mode.

Appropriate homeopathic prescription will not just cure the patient; it will also bring them to a much healthier status than before their illness started.

So, what then can be expected from homeopathy?

Expect from homeopathy that it is a very powerful practice of medicine that can make a big difference in the disease management of the patient whatever the complaint. In some cases this can be obtained very easily and rapidly, in other cases it can take many consultations before the homeopath finds the best possible remedy. The particular conditions that need to be fulfilled to obtain good homeopathic prescription have as a consequence that, in some cases, no satisfying remedy is ever found.

Often, finding the most appropriate remedy is achieved after more than one consultation. Little by little, practitioner and patient make progress along the road of recovery. This often takes the form of a step-by-step improvement with its intermediate aggravations and is the reason why practitioners so often speak of the concept of healing through 'the peeling of the onion'. The road to improvement takes this aspect only because it can take the practitioner some time before he achieves the most appropriate prescription. In the meantime patients may have benefited from prescriptions that only brought temporary or partial success. When at last the most appropriate remedy is found it looks as if the patient has been cured layer by layer. The cure by peeling of the layers should never be the aim of homeopathic prescription; it is only the consequence of the difficulty of successful classical homeopathy.

Luckily, patients can indeed benefit from reasonable good prescriptions that help them through their life and disease without ever enjoying the perfectly, deep and long acting homeopathic remedy.

Always remember that homeopathy is a technique that describes how to find the diluted remedies to which the patient is sensitive. Homeopathy does not explain disease and homeopathic remedies do not have indications for named afflictions or diseases.

The purpose of good classical homeopathic prescription is not to eliminate symptoms but to trigger a smooth and silent reaction in patients that will result in the reduction/elimination of their diseases and therefore their symptoms. The symptoms are the signs of their disease. It is the expression of their disease that should be targeted not the symptoms. The best possible prescription will cure the patient without any spectacular appearances; the patient just gets better and better. The notion that disease comes to the surface causing unusual symptoms to appear in the patient 'while he gets better' and 'eliminates his toxins' is not acceptable. Any respectable homeopath will consider this as being the result of inadequate prescription. It is always possible to do better and that should be the goal.

Practising homeopathy is a humble occupation that often rewards patient and practitioner for the effort they put into the pursuit of its principles.

The practice of homeopathic medicine is fascinating. It is fascinating for its effectiveness and it is fascinating for its view on disease and illness. It is also very demanding. Continuous study and exchange with colleagues is required and there is no place for reflex prescription. Every case is a new case.

In our modern world where logic and common sense are the forces that decide on opinions and tradition, conventional medicine is a few lengths in advance of homeopathy as to what is expected from medical practitioners. It is unlikely that homeopathy will soon become mainstream. There is no efficient (financial) lobby that will ever push it through to the importance it could take in medicine for all. The importance of its presence in the future will be decided by the quality of prescription offered by practitioners and support from health consumers.

When choosing homeopathy, the health consumer takes a bigger part in the decision on treatment strategy than with conventional medicine.

I wish you the best of health for yourself and they that you care about, may homeopathy be on your side when needed.

Preface To The Fifth Edition Of The Organon.

The following is a translation of Hahnemann's introduction to the 5th edition of the Organon. The text is an indication of his thoughts and opinions on the practice of medicine and helps in understanding his motivations that resulted in his principles of homeopathy.

IN order to give a general notion of the treatment of diseases pursued by the old school of medicine (allopathy), I may observe that it presupposes the existence sometimes of excess of blood (plethora which is never present), sometimes of morbid matters and acridities; hence it taps off the life's blood and exerts itself either to clear away the imaginary disease-matter or to conduct it elsewhere (by emetics, purgatives, diuretics, drawing plasters, issues, &c.), in the vain belief that the disease will thereby be weakened and materially eradicated; in place of which the patient's sufferings are thereby increased, and by such and other painful appliances the forces and nutritious juices indispensable to the curative process are abstracted from the organism.

It assails the body with large doses of powerful medicines, often repeated in rapid succession for a long time, whose long-enduring, not infrequently frightful effects it knows not, and which it, purposely it would almost seem, makes unrecognisable by the commingling of several such unknown substances in one prescription, and by their long-continued employment it develops in the body new and often ineradicable medicinal diseases. Whenever it can, it employs, in order to keep in favour with its patient, remedies that immediately suppress and hide the morbid symptoms by opposition for a short time (palliatives), but that leave the disposition to these symptoms (the disease itself) strengthened and aggravated.

It considers symptoms on the exterior of the body as purely local and existing there independently, and vainly supposes that it has cured them when it has driven them away by means of external remedies, so that the internal diseases is thereby compelled to break out on a nobler and more important part. When it knows not what else to do for the disease which will not yield or which grows worse, the old school of medicine undertakes to change it into something else, it knows not what, by means of an alterative, - for example, by the life-undermining calomel, corrosive sublimate and other mercurial preparations in large doses.

The experienced allopath delights to invent a fixed name, by preference a Greek one, for the malady, in order to make the patient believe that he has long known this disease as an old acquaintance, and hence is the fittest person to cure it.

To render (through ignorance) if not fatal, at all events incurable, the vast majority (99/100) of all diseases, namely, those of a chronic character, by continually weakening and tormenting the debilitated patient, already suffering without that from his disease and by adding new destructive drug diseases, this clearly seems to be the unhallowed main business of the old school of medicine (allopathy) - and a very easy business it is when once one has become an adept in this pernicious practice, and is sufficiently insensible to the stings of conscience!

And yet for all these mischievous operations the ordinary physician of the old school can assign his reasons, which, however, rest only on foregone conclusions of his books and teachers, and on the authority of this or that distinguished physician of the old school. Even the most opposite and the most senseless modes of treatment find there their defense, their authority - let their disastrous effects speak ever so loudly against them. It is only under the old physician who has been at last gradually convinced, after many years of misdeeds, of the mischievous nature of his so-called art, and who no longer treats even the severest diseases with anything stronger than plantain water mixed with strawberry syrup (i.e. with nothing), that the smallest number are injured and die.

This non-healing art, which for many centuries has been firmly established in full possession of the power to dispose of the life and death of patients according to its own good will and pleasure, and in that period has shortened the lives of ten times as many human beings as the most destructive wars, and rendered many millions of patients more diseased and wretched than they were originally - this allopathy, I shall first expose somewhat more minutely before teaching in detail its exact opposite, the newly discovered true healing art.

As regards the latter (homeopathy) it is quite otherwise. It can easily convince every reflecting person that the diseases of man are not caused by any substance, any acridity, that is to say, any disease-matter, but that they are solely spirit-like (dynamic) derangements of the spirit-like power (the vital force) that animates the human body. Homeopathy knows that a cure can only take place by the reaction of the vital force against the rightly chosen remedy that has been ingested, and that the cure will be certain and rapid in proportion to the strength with which the vital force still prevails in the patient.

Hence homeopathy avoids everything in the slightest degree enfeebling, and as much as possible every excitation of pain, for pain also diminishes the strength, and hence it employs for the cure ONLY those medicines whose effects in altering and deranging (dynamically) the health it knows accurately, and from these it selects one whose poisoning power (its medicinal disease) is capable of removing the natural disease in question by similarity (similia similibus), and this it administers to the patient in simple form, but in rare and minute doses (so small that, without occasioning pain or weakening, they just suffice to remove the natural malady by means of the reacting energy of the vital force), with this result: that without weakening, injuring or torturing him in the very least, the natural disease is extinguished, and the patient, even whilst he is getting better, gains in strength and thus is cured - an apparently easy but actually troublesome and difficult business, and one requiring much thought, but which restores the patient without suffering in a short time to perfect health, - and thus it is a salutary and blessed business.

Homeopathy sheds not a drop of blood, administers no emetics, purgatives, laxatives or diaphoretics, drives off no external by external means, prescribes no warm baths or medicated clysters, applies no

Spanish flies or mustard plasters, no issues, excites no salivating, burns not with cauterising agents or red-hot iron to the very bone, and so forth, but gives with its own hand its own preparations of simple uncompounded medicines, which it is accurately acquainted with, never subdues pain by opium, etc.

Thus homeopathy is a perfectly simple system of medicine, remaining always fixed in its principles as in its practice, which, like the doctrine whereon it is based, if rightly apprehended will be found to be so exclusive (and only in that way serviceable), that as the doctrine must be accepted in its purity, so it must be purely practised, and all backward straying to the pernicious routine of the old school (whose opposite it is, as day to night) is totally inadmissible, otherwise it ceases to deserve the honorable name of homeopathy.

"I am sorry that I once gave the advice, savouring of allopathy, to apply to the back in psoric diseases a resinous plaster to cause itching, and to employ the finest electrical sparks in paralytic affections. For as both these appliances have seldom proved of service, and have furnished the mongrel homeopaths with an excuse for their allopathic transgressions, I am grieved I should ever have proposed them, and I hereby politely retract them - for this reason also, that, since then, our homeopathic system has advanced so near to perfection that they are now no longer required."

That some misguided physicians who would wish to be considered homoeopathists, engraft some, to them more familiar, allopathic malpractices upon their nominally homeopathic treatment, is owing to ignorance of the doctrine, laziness, contempt for suffering humanity, and ridiculous conceit, and, besides showing unpardonable: negligence in searching for the best homeopathic specific for each case of disease, has often a base love of gain and other sordid motives for its spring - and for its result? That they cannot cure all important and serious diseases (which pure and careful homeopathy can), and that they send many of their patients to that place whence no one returns, whilst the friends console themselves with the reflection that everything (including very hurtful allopathic process!) has been done for the departed.

SAMUEL HAHNEMANN

KOTHEN; March 28th, 1833

Homeopathy from day to day.

It may be stimulating to discover the theory and history behind homeopathic medicine but what really keeps homeopathy alive are the successful cases that occur every day.

What follows is a collection of real clinical cases published by 17 veterinary practitioners. They are often a pleasure to read and are examples of the reality behind daily practice of classical homeopathy. Cases, like the ones below, have been published because the improvement in each of them was most certainly linked to the administration of the homeopathic remedy and followed the rules for holistic improvement. This means that it was obvious that the disease or complaint was eliminated efficiently without being replaced by another complaint and this for a sufficiently long time to ascertain that the remedy was homeopathic to the patient. In some cases the feedback is short but the spectacular type of improvement (or particular type of patient) then usually justifies publication. The other reason for their publication is the didactic value they have; they may highlight an original aspect of a remedy, an original remedy selection process, an illustration of the tenacity that is sometimes needed before the patient benefits or merely be an example of good remedy selection technique.

Such examples help the homeopathic community to exchange ideas and improve prescription. The advantage of having cases of several authors brought together is that what is shown here is not the product of the imagination or opinion of one person.

The authors of the various cases are all homeopaths who apply classical prescription. None of the cases has been made up: they are all genuine. I know the authors well enough to guarantee authenticity. None of them are pure homeopaths; they all are in conventional practice but make efforts to show and explain to their clients why it is wise to choose homeopathy as one of the better treatment options, by exercising high standard homeopathic prescription. If other medicines were used at the same time this is mentioned.

Some of the cases date from 20 years ago, others are more recent. As a consequence there is some variability in the attitude of the practitioner between the different case records; classical homeopathic prescription has

101

changed and progressed enormously over the last twenty years. In a few cases, practitioners themselves comment how unsatisfactory their previous prescriptions were.

You will discover new aspects to remedies that seem familiar. Although some cases will be followed by general comments, it is not intended to propose remedy snapshots for prescription. Homeopathy should not be learned from one publication; it is best learned in an open minded well-organised supportive teaching course that will take many years and probably a life-time.

There are simple cases and complicated ones, cases that found a quick solution and others where clients have been very patient. The most common technique used to select remedies is through repertorising. This is a technique where the homeopath lines up several symptoms that are considered homeopathic to the case to see what remedy (or remedies) is (are) covered by these symptoms.

For this purpose we use a repertory, which is a book (or computer program) that lines up thousands of symptoms classified per body function where they apply, followed by all the remedies that are associated with each symptom. Cross matching indicates possible remedies. Knowledge of remedies helps to select the most appropriate one in the light of the atmosphere of the case. Sometimes remedies are selected based on one symptom only. In other cases selection was based on the supposed knowledge of a remedy picture. You will see that this system is not always the most reliable one.

The cases where clients have been very patient are proof that it is not always necessary to have instant results in medicine; the instant result culture of our modern times is often a barrier to sensible medicine. Modern medicine has a tendency to 'blast' away symptoms in order to please the client/patient. Blasting away symptoms may be much appreciated but does not always make the patient happy (in the long term). Many chronic diseases can be attributed to aggressive suppression of symptoms.

Unless there is a real emergency (not very common), many cases (acute and chronic) can be dealt with patiently. Certainly in homeopathy this patience is often rewarded with a positive outcome. Patience is ly needed to allow the homeopath to arrive at the adequate conclusion. Once a really appropriate remedy is found for the patient, its activity is in the majority of cases surprisingly fast.

The cases are more or less summarised. Sometimes efforts are made to edit them into readable stories. Even then they reflect how the homeopath receives the information on his patient. You will discover how the stories sometimes jump from one subject to another and even contain contradictions. Everything that is said (or observed) about a patient can have its importance; Hahnemann showed the importance of this when he compiled the symptoms observed during remedy testing and when he stressed how important it was to see the patient as an individual.

When texts reproduce the client's words, this is indicated by the ' ' signs. It is up to the homeopath to find what is important in each story that can be used to select a remedy. Never should an owner of an animal be accused of inconsistency when they seem to give contradictory observations in the same or consequent consultations. Very often there is a good explanation for this in the light of the case.

In some cases authors made interpretations that may look unscientific or risky. They are mostly justified by the context or atmosphere of the consultation. Such an atmosphere is difficult to reproduce in a written text.

Becoming an experienced homeopath is learning how to use symptoms and observations successfully. In the absence of comments made by our patients (animals) we have to work with the material that is offered to us. A little bit of interpretation can be very helpful if it is used sensibly. This is the part of homeopathy that is more Art than Science. Even in conventional medicine the Art of medical practice is usually of great benefit to patients. Pure science is insufficient to cover the infinite number of different problems that the patients present to their doctors and vets.

In several cases one could be justified in observing that the 'patients' haven't been particularly well trained. In most of these cases, an appropriate homeopathic prescription improves the animal's behaviour (as well as the original complaint) without the need for severe corrections; following the remedy, animals tend to take less advantage from the failings in training with, as a result, better harmony in the 'family'

With regards to training , it is my observation that many animals that are very strictly trained cannot express themselves sufficiently. This translates often into chronic re-occurring physical problems to which no real solutions are found with conventional medicine. Homeopathy can help in these cases but only if the owners or keepers are open-minded enough to request homeopathic prescription and talk to the consultant in an open spontaneous manner without being afraid of sounding ridiculous. In homeopathic medicine, no observation is absurd, especially not when it is spontaneous. Never try to be scientific if you talk to a homeopath; this will often diminish the value of the information

The titles of the cases refer to certain aspects of the remedy or an important central point of the case or homeopathy in general. The names of the animals have been changed.

You will meet dogs and cats, horses and cattle and there are even a few feathers that will come on the stage to enlighten you about their brilliant recoveries. Discover the power of the singular homeopathic remedy and enjoy the reading!

And from some of the histories you may learn that your pet is not the worst in the world.

(Full names and addresses of the authors can be found on page 269.)

1) When you are called Tiger you are a cool cat. (M. Brunson)

Tiger is a tall, castrated, 4 year old tom cat. Eight days ago he had an unfortunate encounter with a car and broke his femur. Orthopaedic surgery was performed to repair the broken femur with a pin.

He does not recuperate well from the surgery. He walks on his leg but he continues to have a temperature even though he receives daily antibiotics. He doesn't eat and he drinks more. He stays on the bed, as usual a little isolated from his owners; he prefers the bedroom upstairs.

When he arrives in the surgery he has a look around and then settles down on a wiping cloth that was left rather central in the room.

Usually he eats well but does not put on weight easily.

Why not use Arnica? This case is the obvious consequence of a double traumatism: accident and surgery.

The vet noticed that the owner talks about Tiger as if he is his usual self, as if the traumas haven't made a big difference in the way he reacts. He therefore decides to use Tiger's general symptoms to search for an appropriate remedy.

Natrum muriaticum 30C is administered twice. The selection of the remedy was based on a first impression.

The next day Tiger is back in the consulting room. The remedy has not made any difference.

The vet asks for some more information about the patient.

His owner comments: "He is not a cuddly cat, he does not really like to stay on our knees. He often disappears for long periods and generally sleeps upstairs where it is quiet. Usually he drinks little and he doesn't like milk. He goes out as much in the winter as during the summer."

This time, Tiger chooses to settle himself comfortably in the chair next to his owner.

Based on aversion to milk and prefers to be on his own, Sulfur is selected as a remedy because of the relaxed attitude of this cat (goes out a lot, and settles comfortably in a chair in the vets surgery or, previously, in the middle of the consult room on a wiping cloth). Also, Sulfur is present in 'appetite wanting with thirst'.

Three granules (30C potency) in the evening and three in the morning and all settles within 24 hours.

This is a nice example to show that Sulfur is not just a 'skin remedy'. As long as the patient corresponds to the dynamics of this remedy it can do a lot of things: check the following case!

2) I am not called Tiger, but I am certainly cool. (E. De Beukelaer)

Helios is a 5 year old gelding of unknown origin. He suffers from a condition called Wobbler syndrome. This condition was diagnosed at the veterinary faculty in Paris. As a consequence Helios has a lack of coordination and weakness in his hind legs (this is caused by pressure on the spinal chord in the neck region). Helios can walk slowly but when he tries to have a gallop in his field, he staggers like a drunk and regularly slips and falls over.

When I meet him for the first time, he is lying in a deep ditch on his side in the water, his legs tangled in roots and branches. He lies there quietly and helplessly.

After a shot of painkillers and with the help of a digger, strong ropes and the fire brigade, we manage to pull him from his awkward position two metres upwards on to a nice straw bed that had been prepared on the side. All of this happens in a very quiet atmosphere, no panicking of the horse, no need for sedation, which is rather unusual.

In the afternoon, when I went out to check on him, the straw bed was abandoned; he was already transported five miles further to his owner's house and was enjoying a nice meal. No obvious signs visible of his experience. Helios is certainly cool!

His owner tells me about his handicap that was probably the cause of his fall in the river. Together we decide to try and do something about his problem by using homeopathy. (The faculty in Paris had given no hope as to the outcome of the case.)

I noted the following interesting points during this first consultation:
- he has been very itchy this summer and scratching has been a major difficulty because of his handicap.
- his neck has always been stiff and produces cracking noises from time to time.
- he does not like to walk in puddles, he goes around them.
- he likes being brushed and will stand for hours, otherwise he is inconsiderate to us, he is curious and pushes us away as if we were not there.
- sometimes he seems anxious.
- 'time goes by' says his owner referring to his attitude.
- he was a big foal, his birth was laborious, he had a long neck like a giraffe.
- he always has been the boss over the other foal. He tried with us but soon found out that that didn't work. His owners have to keep on reminding him.
- he is difficult to feed, he does not put on weight very easily.
- he often has passages of mild diarrhoea that go away without treatment.

A first prescription is of Natrum carbonicum is made, based on: cracking in the neck region , rubbing ameliorates , aversion to wetting of feet.

No change in the next three weeks; wrong remedy.

When I speak to the owner again three weeks later he adds that Helios likes the salt lick and that since his illness, he has become 'nicer'. They refer to him as 'the junky' because of his placid attitude.

I add the following symptoms to my search: desire for salt, lean, tottering gait, as in if a dream.

107

The only remedy present is Sulfur: one 200k dose solves his hind leg paresis in three weeks time. Four years later his owners still ride him without the need for any further prescriptions.

3) A classic but effective prescription. (M. Brunson)

A small, 12 weeks old puppy is presented for severe diarrhoea. He vomits all he drinks. His stools are very watery and brown in colour. After having vomited, he hides behind the settee. He continues to eat. He feels the cold and trembles when he goes out. He changes place all the time and does not want to be left alone.

In the consultation room he seems indifferent to everything. His temperature is normal, his eyes are dirty and his nose is cold right up to the bone.

Desire to hide, coldness of nose, worse when alone, restlessness driving from place to place point to Arsenicum album. This looks like a remedy that fits the picture but there is no change in 24 hours after three administrations of the 30C potency.

In such acute cases it is necessary to change remedy rapidly if the initial choice does not seem to have the desired effect.

A second symptom selection using worse when alone, indifference to everything and appetite during heat, indicate Phosphorus. Two 30k doses solve the case in a few hours.

In this case the usual remedy picture of Arsenicum album seemed much more applicable than the picture of Phosphorus. Such cases are a nice indication that the patient knows better then the homeopathic community. It is the patient who decides upon the treatment not the tradition of the homeopath. Some homeopaths may say that there is a blockage because the patient does not react to the appropriate remedy... hmm, could be patronising?

4) Caring but weary! (M. Brunson)

Kitty is a little 5.5 months old kitten. Rather small for her age she is the smallest of the litter. She has recurring cat flu resulting in the production of a bilateral thick discharge from her eyes. These symptoms appeared for the first time when she was only a few weeks old.

"She is always full of life, never discommoded by her chronic disease. Although she is small, she is very adventurous and protects another kitten that lives in the house. When this one goes out too far she brings it back to a safe place. She is always out and about on her own."
She does not stay in the owner's arms that much any more. Cuddling is not her favourite pastime. She will wiggle until she is freed from their arms.

"She likes looking out of the window where she always seems ready for action. The flies have a rough time and don't know where to hide. She likes to sit in high places.

She is very caring towards the other kitten, which is allowed to eat out of her dish and sleep on her legs. Kitty doesn't like to be taken care of: she will fight and jump out of our arms. She is intelligent, attentive and agile.

She is very cautious when new situations occur, she is startled by noise. She sleeps against the hot radiator. She likes all dairy products but will not eat anything else from our table. She is not a big eater."

The image that radiates from the case seems to make it a classical indication for the prescription of Nux vomica. She receives two 30C doses but the remedy produces no result at all.

Kitty is presented again three weeks later.
When she enters the consulting room she shoots through the door, has a good run around and installs herself at the window where she observes with great interest all that happens outside.

Sneezing continues.

"She is still very bouncy, she continues to take care of the other kitten, which is not allowed to go outside. She does not like to be taken in our arms and claws to free herself. She still loves the hot radiator."

The following symptoms are used: Vivacious, anxiety for others, heedless, warm stove ameliorates, nose purulent discharge.
Kitty receives Hepar sulfur 30K once. She got worse for a few days and then the chronic disease cleared.

Six months later she has a blocked nose again. The same remedy is repeated with the same rapid result. No further prescription has been necessary.

Hepar sulfur is more than a remedy for control and treatment of abscesses and suppuration. It has a picture of its own. Vulnerability is quite central, whether one considers oneself vulnerable (Kitty did not want to be held in the arms) or whether one is sensitive to the vulnerability of others (Kitty protects the other kitten).

5) I am supposed to be a guard dog but I am afraid of the dark. (B Heude)

Phenix is afraid of everything. He is supposed to guard the house to comfort his lady owner but he runs off as soon as there is any danger. He is rather wild. He hides in the bathroom when he hears a noise. He is afraid of the neighbours, the son and the brother in law, even though they visit regularly. Nobody can approach him.
Will he ever become the guard dog he is supposed to be?

This sort of condition is well recognised and is caused by a lack of contact with the real world before the age of two months (kenneled inside a building). Usually things are aggravated by an abrupt introduction into the real world (transport to shop and then new owner). The result is a frightened puppy incapable of adapting to any new circumstances and constantly anxious. For a Belgian shepherd (Groenendael) with a nervous race disposition, Phenix had a very unfortunate start in life resulting in his failure to become the dog he was expected to be.

Phenix is two when he is presented to the homeopathic vet.

In the surgery he is absolutely petrified and tries to hide behind the chair. He tries to explore a little but every time fear overcomes him and he retreats to his hiding place.

"When we bought him in the shop, the shopkeeper picked him up by the skin of the neck and plunged him into the boot of our car (!). On the way home he vomited and we stopped the car because it urgently needed a clean up. There was a big struggle to put his collar on. Once outside the car, Phenix wiggled so much that he slipped out of the collar and ran off into the village where we were parked, risking a car accident at any time.
After a major search operation helped by many villagers, we found him hiding in the cellar of a house where we finally managed to catch him.
Arrived home, he took refuge behind the boiler, only to reappear at night to eat his food. It has taken me 15 days before I could approach him. I am now the only person he trusts. It has taken me a long time. It is still impossible to go out with him in town."

The plan is to find a homeopathic remedy to overcome as much of his anxiety as possible to start a (re) training program. Phenix is already too old to expect full recovery but that shouldn't be a reason not to give him a good chance for improvement. (There is always a possibility of achieving results if the right effort is delivered.)

The owner makes further comments on his behaviour:
" He is very attached to me, he follows me wherever I go. He waits for my approval before he does anything. He chews everything that lies around. Everything he finds gets ripped to pieces. He is a very lovable dog.
It has taken a long time before he risked going out in the garden when it was dark: he stayed in the places that were lit by the lanterns. In

the house he is scared of light reflections (mirror): he growls and his fur comes up. I have to talk to him and stroke him to calm him. The next day it starts all over again: he does not seem to learn."

Phenix' fear of the dark is an unusual observation. In cases like his where dogs suffer from a lack of socialisation, they tend to prefer to hide in the dark. The owner's comments about his fear of reflected light is also unusual.

Phenix goes home with one dose of Stramonium 1M and some essential basic advice on how to teach him to stand up for himself.

Second visit three months later.
He has made great progress: no more fear of the dark, no more fear of reflections and he follows the son when he goes out jogging. He still finds it difficult to go out in town: this is normal and will be the next stage of his acclimatisation.
Phenix is given a new dose of Stramonium, this time 10M dilution and some further advice on how to introduce him little by little to go into town.

Third visit two months later:
Phenix now goes out in town on the lead like a normal dog. He is just wary when big lorries or motorbikes drive by but his behaviour is controllable.

The owner also complained about two other problems: lack of desire to obey his owner's orders and the impression of aggressiveness to other dogs. This behaviour was mostly due to the owner's kindness. To appease him she was always trying to comfort him. Dogs tend to read in this human behaviour a different message from the one we want to send them. It often increases their anxiety because they think we sense a danger or conflict situation. The owner in this case was too wary to let him approach any other dogs out of fear of fights. This resulted (like it usually does) in fierce barking behaviour when Phenix crossed any strange dogs.

After having received further advice, Phenix' owner has become firmer and more relaxed about other dogs. Although Phenix still gets away with lots of things, his behaviour is as good as it can be. The remaining problems cannot be solved with homeopathic treatment because they are 'normal' in the light of the relationship in the 'family'. Homeopathy allowed Phenix to behave normally; normal reactions to conflict situations and normal reactions to his owner's attitude. This attitude was rather lenient resulting in a behaviour that is not perfectly by the book. What homeopathy does achieve is that after having received an appropriate homeopathic remedy, animals usually take less advantage of easygoing owners.

6) I am not afraid but lost my 'place'. (E. De Beukelaer)

Sam is an 8 year old Siamese cat. He has never been ill until one day he develops kidney failure. He stopped eating, started drinking more, lost weight. On a blood sample his kidney values (urea and creatinine) are way above normal. Classic conventional treatment for 10 days does not make any difference. He gets worse and worse and now his kidney values are so high that euthanasia is considered; his kidney failure seems obviously irreversible.

Sam is not suffering, he still has a sparkle in his eyes; I ask for 48 hours delay to give him the chance to benefit from a homeopathic prescription.

The owner is asked to tell Sam's story because the clinical symptoms he presents are those normally associated with kidney failure and therefore are of no benefit for the selection of a homeopathic remedy.

"He hides everywhere; he doesn't seem to like men anymore. He was the best friend of my son and now when my son comes in the house, he flees. He always has been easily frightened. He has a terrified look on him. He drinks large quantities of water.

Three years ago a third cat joined the family. At first Sam was upset but then he accepted that the new cat, which was a little bullish, took an important position in the pecking order. Sam's place was reduced from second to third.

Since a few weeks ago, he doesn't want to jump up onto his normal sleeping places anymore. He calls us to help him but sometimes he jumps up there behind our back. Outside he spends his time sitting in the middle of the flowerbed and moves away when we or the other cats approach. He sometimes stays there in the cold and the rain. Normally he used not to go out a lot. He never liked to be carried but now asks to be picked up.

He used to eat anything. He has always been slightly picked on by the other cat; he now shrinks away when he approaches. Sometimes he complains when you lift him up. He doesn't come up to our bed anymore in the morning; it used to be a religion. He was always a little jumpy to noise and afraid of strangers; he never got used to the cleaning lady (after 7 years)."

The homeopathic symptoms retained are;

Fear of being approached, does not recognise his relatives, feeling of helplessness, thirst large quantities (this was a less 'homeopathic' symptom but thought to be helpful in confirming the remedy)

Phosphorus and Stramonium both present these four symptoms.

If the notion of his aversion for strangers is added, Stramonium is most indicated. Also the unusual behaviour of sitting outside in the flowerbed, in the cold and rain tend to confirm this remedy.

Stramonium 30K is administered twice per day for two days. The second day Sam becomes interested in food again. The remedy is stopped and Sam continues to improve. A week later he receives a further dose of the same remedy because the improvement seems to stagnate.

A week further, he has put most of his weight back on and enjoys the company of the oldest son in the house again.
For three months Sam is his back to his usual self.

When I see him again, the owners had just collected him from the kennels where he stayed during the family holiday. Nobody in the cattery had noticed he wasn't eating. His kidneys must have collapsed again and he is a dying cat. He is put to sleep by my colleague.

Sam's owners were still very pleased with the results of the homeopathic prescription. Maybe I should have pressed them to come for follow up visits soon after Sam's improvement. Maybe further administrations of the remedy (or a different remedy if the interrogation and blood results would have suggested this) could have helped Sam to continue to overcome his illness.

It is common to see that when homeopathy delivered unexpected results in cases that are conventionally considered to be lost, clients just enjoy the results without realising that further intervention may be possible. We are so conditioned by prognosis based only on what conventional medicine is capable of making happen, that we find it difficult to imagine that there are other options that may be more successful.

This is an interesting case because this remedy is mostly associated with 'wild behaviour'. Sam was not wild: he 'lost his place': from the interrogation I sensed that Sam had never really overcome the arrival of the new cat that had pushed him down the pecking order.

7) And in the farmyard...   (A. Duport)

The vet is called out for a calf born the day before. The farmer had left it a little late to help the cow give birth and her calf has suffered from a lack of oxygen. This lack of oxygen has affected the calf; he cannot stand up and finds it difficult to lift his head. Also his lungs are filled with amniotic fluid; 'he drowned in his water' as this is usually described. In a farmyard these cases have a poor prognosis; therefore efficient medicine is required.

The vet observes the following: the calf has dragged himself to the side of the stable, his jaws are clenched together, his legs are cold and his tongue is drawn backwards in his mouth. There is no sucking reflex when the vet puts his finger in his (the calf's!) mouth and he bellows (not the vet) when moved around. He doesn't even react when a little milk is poured in his mouth.

The farmer told him that mother cow was very 'stressed' when she was moved from the field to the stable after the calving. She has adopted the calf normally. It is now impossible to approach her and she kicks in all directions when the farmer and vet come close to her.

The vet chooses the following symptoms: Jaws clenched together, lack of reaction and fear of strangers (symptoms very strongly present with the mother and also with the calf).
Ambra grisea is selected and given to calf and cow. This is followed by a rapid improvement over a period of 2 days. Calf and cow both returned to normal.

It such early life situations, the symptoms of mother and baby can be combined in the selection for an appropriate remedy.

8) Control takes over. (M. Brunson)

Caesar loses blood from his urethra opening. Drops of blood colour the flooring in the house on a regular basis. This has been going on for more then a year. His prostate, bladder and all the rest of his urinary tract has been examined from all angles but no diagnosis could be made. When it starts, its lasts for a few days, Caesar has two to three occurrences per month.

He is an active 6 year old Dachshund who controls the whole family.

He bleeds the most at night, when he plays and when he is alone.

"We are his slaves; we have to take care of him all the time; he is always under my feet; he drives me mad.

Things got worse when we stopped taking him to work. He is very affectionate but over-attached to us.

He contracts his back very often: two to three times per month. If he is outside it goes away by itself very quickly, if he is inside with me it takes much longer to go away. It has been happening less often lately but then he had more bleeding problems.

He always smiles at everybody.

If we leave him at the kennels he is fine. He is a comedian; his problems come when we are around. He is not clean at night. He trembles all the time because he is afraid that we abandon him. He always wants to be perfect. He has no existence by himself. If we laugh at him he is hurt and sulks."

Pulsatilla 200K makes no difference

One month later;

He is certainly not better; on two occasions he bled large amounts instead of the usual dribble. He also produced a few clots at some point.

Secale cornutum 30C twice per day for two days brings an improvement.

Two weeks later:

"He is worse when my husband is there. When he is in the kennels, there is no problem. We went on holiday to the seaside; when we left him alone in the apartment he caused a lot of damage."

Secale c. is repeated in XMK once.

He becomes livelier and bleeds less.

Two months later.

He is still not right; the following remark of the owner shows that previous prescription was suppressive: "He is an unhappy dog." There is less bleeding but mentally he is less well; this is an aggravation of the patient.

"He loves children and especially babies; he licks them all over. He is always busy and always under our feet."

China 200K: no change

Two weeks later: Carcinosine 200K; no change
Later again: Phosphorus 200K: no change.

The owners consult a colleague who castrates the dog.

He comes back two months later because following the castration things got worse.

The clients repeat the same story: " He is better in the kennels, he controls us. He is always busy. He loves children"

It is now time to sit back and discover what motivates the dog's behaviour.

He is always active and takes in all the space in the house; he is invading. It does not seem so much that he is dependant on his owners (OK when in kennels) but that he wants to control them.

This notion of invasion, keeping in control suggests Lyssinum as a remedy (the nosode of Rabies)

He receives one dose of Lyssinum 200K.

Following the remedy, his troubles disappear and he finally starts to behave like a normal dog. He still loves his family but he can keep his distance from them; he has given up being a slave master. (It is interesting at this point to look again at the exact words of the owners in the first consultation; they really express how the dog 'controls' the owners and how his behaviour is 'controlled' by their presence.)

It is common that in unsuccessful cases, given the opportunity, good prescription can be achieved if the practitioner is given the chance to sit back and discover the theme that runs through the various consultations. This demands time and effort from the client but helps in finding solutions where uncommon remedies are required.

9) I am tough but fragile. (J Dabeux)

Sage is a 7 year old collie cross bitch who is presented for dry fur and large, non-itchy, bald patches all over her body. The owner is not interested in a diagnosis; he doesn't want complementary examinations to be performed. He wants a treatment to improve his bitch.

The vet explains that homeopathy would be a sensible option and asks him to talk about his dog.

"She seems to have aged, she has lost her usual energy. This has started after her first and only litter two years ago. One day, when I arrived from work, she had her tail between her legs and was as if paralysed. Since then she hasn't jumped in the car anymore and her breath has become very smelly. She doesn't greet me anymore when I come home in the evening.

From her litter we kept one pup. She took very good care of it and she has always been dominant over it until lately. First her coat has become dry and then she started to lose hair in different places. There was never any itching. She has become disinterested in her daughter who has now taken over the dominant role and eats out of her bowl.

She was spayed a year ago. She was a normal pup and always has been a very energetic dog.

Sage was easy to train and is very obedient. She liked the agility training and worked hard. She is very sport minded and likes to run fast. When she hurts herself (which happens from time to time because of all her running) she retreats into a corner, doesn't complain and does not want to be touched. She has a dominant character and is as stubborn as anything!

When we call her she comes to us as if she wants to do us a service, which pleases her. She is a glutton and has stolen food from the table (even vegetables). She does not like to be wet and likes her comfort: she wants her blanket to lie on and never lies on the floor. She always has bad breath. Her seasons come regularly with normal blood loss. She eats anything even other dog's droppings!

She is a tough one but at the same time very sensitive and fragile."

The homeopathic symptoms used for repertorisation are:
Aversion to be touched, headstrong, industrious, putrid odor from mouth, complaints after delivery and says is well when very sick.

Arnica 30C is given twice per day for three days. Two weeks later the fur starts to grow back and she regains authority over her daughter. She receives one further 200K dose of Arnica after three weeks.

Three months later her skin is back to normal, she still finds it a little difficult to jump into the car. She then receives another dose of Arnica 200K and everything returns to normal in a few weeks time.

Two years later she is still fine.
This is one of the many examples that show that Arnica is more then a remedy for bruises and other traumas when proper classical prescription technique is applied!

10) I should be important. (P Rouchossé)

This old gun dog 'arrived' by himself one day, 6 months earlier at the client's house and settled in. He still has no name and is called 'The Dog'. Since a few days ago he cannot run anymore, he stops and has to lie down. On auscultation there is an significant cardiac arrhythmia with extra systoles. X rays show an enlarged heart; 'The Dog' suffers from severe heart failure.

The owner explains:
"He does not finish his dish, he is scared, he is a scared dog. He growls at other dogs but runs away. He is very dignified; one could even say 'haughty'.
He does not like to be on his own but sometimes disappears for two or three days. He cannot stand to be locked in: he will do whatever he can to get out. He overturns his bowl to eat his food from the ground.
He growls at bearded old people. One day he completely wrecked the broom; we think that a bearded person must have hit him with a broom.
He growls at people that are unpleasant to me. Nobody is allowed to do any harm to my family or me. He is contradictory: sometimes full of life and sometimes without energy. He just does what he wants. He growls at people behind the gate but when they enter he runs off to his bed: he doesn't like anybody to come into his territory but he is rather cowardly.
Sometimes he gives the impression that death is near.

When I punish him, he doesn't eat for three days. He punishes himself. He is a rambler"

The impression the dog gives to the vet is both dignity and sadness. He has very clean teeth but has a very old look about him. His age is not known. He has crusty growths on his eyelids.

The vet asks: 'How is he with females?'

"When he has adopted a bitch, she becomes his property. When the other dog is not there he is the boss. He is very possessive and he is selfish.

He never drinks water; he refuses to drink water. He only drinks powdered milk. He eats everything prepared with gravy. He loves sugar; he would do anything for sugar. He drinks coffee, eats chocolate, nuts, eggs and salad.

He acts like a human: he sings in front of the radio, he watches television and pushes on the remote control (!?). In the morning at six, he stops the alarm clock and wakes us. At twelve he goes to the table and calls us.

Everything is appearance with him, unless he gets cross and then he may harm you. If there is a fly in his dish, he will not eat. He growls at people who wear strong fragrances.

My dog is arrogant!

He punishes himself before I punishes him, he wants to be perfect!"

The vet: 'And his sleep?'

"He has his own bed. You cannot take it away: one day I washed it and then he shredded it to pieces. I have given him another one; he takes it everywhere with him. He always sleeps on his back.

He is afraid of water; he will go miles around a puddle. He hates the cold. If we'd keep him in for three days he would hold back from going to the toilet.

He only eats hot food, nearly burning. When it cools down, he pushes his bowl to the kitchen to have his food reheated.

There are some people he hates."

Compared to many cases where one searches desperately for homeopathic symptoms, this case seems to have too many. What symptoms to choose? What is it that makes this dog really original?

The vet's approach was to classify the observations into groups to obtain the following: conscientious about trifles, haughty and cowardly, remorseful and sulky, aversion to water, changeable mood, sensitive to odours, desire for coffee, desire for warm food.

A large number of remedies that have these symptoms/themes in their pathogenesis present themselves as candidates, Aurum has been chosen for the desire to excel: the owner did say that "he thinks he fails in everything and makes many efforts to achieve his goals."

One dose of Aurum met. 9C every two days. The third day his owner rings to say that he is completely changed: no more capriciousness, no more fear of water and excellent physical condition. (He only received two doses.)

One year later he is still fine. In the case of severe heart failure this is quite a remarkable result.

11) When the need is high, homeopathy is nearby. (B Heude)

Bresil, a 12 year old queen, is presented for mouth ulcers and very inflamed pharyngeal gums. She doesn't eat or drink, she is dehydrated and salivates constantly.
The owner does not want homeopathic treatment and antibiotics are dispensed for her.

Two days later, they come back with Bresil who improved only mildly. They also bring two young kittens (aged five months) with ulcers on their tongues. This indicates that there is a viral infection going around in the cat family. The kitten's mouths seem painful and their behaviour is what can be expected normally from ill kittens: not eating, lethargic, temperature: nothing to base a homeopathic prescription on.

One thing attracts the vet's attention: one of the kittens has two perfectly symmetric ulcers on the back of his tongue.

Because of the viral nature (no real effective treatment exists) the owners agree to try a homeopathic remedy.

Kali muriaticum is selected based on the symmetric nature of the ulcers of the one kitten. One administration in 5C at noon and the two kittens start to eat again the same evening.

The client comes back the next day for some of the same granules for Bresil who recuperates in three days with the same remedy.

In such 'epidemic' situations, the same remedy will often treat most individuals in the group, once the original features/symptoms of the 'epidemic' are found and have indicated the appropriate remedy.

12) Not all cases are spectacular and clear, but patients can still benefit. (M. Brunson)

'Oldie' is a 13 year old cross-bred dog. He is presented for coughing.

The cough is dry and rough and started 5 days ago. Previously, he has had two similar passages of coughing; they only lasted for one day.

It is very difficult to listen to his chest, Oldie is a difficult dog: he growls, barks, tries to bite and then starts to cough.

He has recently aged. He refuses to stay on his own; he becomes very destructive when he is on his own. He tries to hide when he is frightened (when alone or when there is a sudden noise). When he goes out he wants to come back in as soon as possible, he always has his tail between his legs, he follows his owner around everywhere.

"He doesn't sleep well anymore; he tosses all the time. He does not obey anymore; he does what he decides.

When he was younger, he was nervous, never satisfied, always whining, going in and going out. He is jealous; he steals the goat's bread to bury it. He is jealous of my wife.

He never liked strangers; he has become indifferent to them. He is excited all day and by 5 pm he goes to sleep. He is quiet for a while and becomes restless again in the night.

Before he had a capricious appetite, now he eats everything and especially craves sweets. He never drinks.

He still wants to be fussed all the time. As soon as the sun comes out he will be sunbathing, in the summer he prefers the shade. He doesn't like extreme temperatures: not too hot not too cold.

Eight years old he was bitten by another dog on his private parts and needed a castration. Over the years he has become afraid of thunder and gunshots: he hides."

Based on the general picture, Lycopodium 30C is given once which resolves the cough in a few hours.

He comes back 18 months later: It is planned that he will spend the holidays with the parents and usually every time he meets their dog he starts to cough. The owner wants a preventative treatment. One dose of Lycopodium 6LM is dispensed.

Five months later.

The holiday period passed without problems but Oldie starts to change: his hearing is going. He is still startled when something falls over or when there are high-pitched noises. It seems that Lycopodium has helped him very well but his ageing process does not show the serenity we would expect after a really homeopathic remedy.

"He always whimpers; he only stops when he lies on the sofa. He cannot find the right place to be. He eats more and does not put on any weight.

A wart has grown on one of the eyelids. His jealous attitude has disappeared. He really suffered from the heat this summer and needed to move from place to place as soon as he became hot.

He drinks often and in large quantities, he yawns, he seems without reaction."

Without making an in-depth analysis, Sulfur 30K is given once.

This dose improves his general state but the remedy has little influence on the coughing that keeps on coming and going over the next few months.

Oldie is presented again eight months later.
"He still drinks large amounts and has lost some weight. He coughs very frequently: he has to get up from his basket and goes outside where the cough improves. He coughs when he gets excited: when we leave the house and come back in the evening.

He has bad wind when he coughs. The wind is worse when he receives tinned food. He now accepts staying on his own, he is ageing, he does not follow the paths in the garden anymore: he goes across without paying attention."

Sulfur 30K is repeated because it gave him a boost of energy for many months last time.

One month later, the cough has become very bad and disturbing. Sulfur is not a good remedy for Oldie. The cough is now worse; it is aggravated at the least cooling of the weather. Any emotions, exercise and drinking make him cough.

"He has become really old, he is becoming senile and dull but he still runs after the cats. He is more scared of thunderstorms than before. He drinks large amounts and continues to lose weight despite his increased appetite. He still does not like to stay on his own but does not always realise that he is on his own."

Phosphorus 30 one dose, based on the knowledge of the remedy.

Well no! After 4 days he is worse. The outside cold really makes his cough much worse.

This time the homeopath takes back the whole file and selects a few symptoms that are sure: emaciation with increase appetite, lack of reaction, cough in old people, cough aggravated by cold.

Psorinum 12C is given with a remarkable result and is repeated in a 30k strength eight days later. He recovers very well and his cough disappears. He is presented a year later (he is now 17!). He has started coughing again.

Psorinum 30K has no effect, Psorinum 6LM a week later puts him back in shape and the cough disappears.

He is seen again three months later and is doing fine. Only the deafness is worse.

He dies peacefully in his sleep six months later.

Only for the selection of the last remedy was the usual homeopathic selection process applied. The author of this case is a well-known and experienced veterinary homeopath and director of a homeopathy school in Belgium. He commented on this case that whatever your experience with remedies, don't just rely on your memory to prescribe them. Take time to analyse the case and use a proper prescription technique to give the patient the best possible chances. (He rarely publishes his brilliant cases. He mostly publishes cases that have an educational value for students and others who are willing to improve, showing pitfalls to try and avoid, original remedy selections or sound basic homeopathic technique.)

Another facet of this case is that patients can benefit from different remedies during their life. Prescription does not always need to be 'perfect' to produce an acceptable result.

13) Step by step one discovers what really drives the patient. (B Heude)

Frizzy is a two year old Angora rabbit. She is a marvel! She arrived at her new house two months ago where she became immediately attached to Dany an eight year old collie bitch whom she considers as her mum. She is also very attached to Duke, one of the many other, male, house rabbits.

Two months after her arrival she develops peculiar behaviour: She starts to pull the fur from her belly, makes a nest and pretends she has babies.

Based on the impression 'delusion she was nursing her child' one dose of Atropinum 30C solves the behaviour in no time.

Two months later, she develops rabbit flu. She sneezes frequently and there is a severe conjunctivitis. The further developments of the case will show that Atropinum solved the temporary symptoms but not Frizzy's chronic problems or underlying 'cause'.
The owner explains:
- she is startled by sudden noises
- when she is stressed during thunderstorms she pulls her fur.
- she fears strangers.
- she gives the impression she guards the house: she sits behind the door and seems to growl when she hears suspected noises.
- she plays like a cat with balls and other cat toys: she will chase them around the house.
- she is spoiled, she receives delicacies: she only accepts the best quality biscuits for people.
- she drinks large amounts and often.
- she does not eat any fruit but thrives on carrots and only will eat curly salad: she urinates on any other salad we give her.
- she does not like the cold, she stays away from doors where the air blows underneath.
- when we reprimand her, she is cross and seems to imagine that we are laughing at her.

One dose of Silicea 9C clears the problems for 2 months. She then relapses and is cured again with a 12C dose but when she rapidly relapses again a further dose of the remedy does not function anymore.

She is presented again (six months later) for a new consultation: her fur has become dull and falls out in certain places. She sneezes frequently and has repeated episodes of diarrhoea. Several allopathic medicines have been used unsuccessfully since the last homeopathic consultation/treatment.
- her mate Duke died two months ago, she has looked for him all over the place, she liked him very much.

- a new mate was bought but she did not like him and stayed away from him.
- she now dislikes the person that looked after her the most (the handicapped child of the family), she will go up to her and bite her when she says something 'wrong'.
- she still loves Dany but she is very jealous towards her, she will push her away and then chases her when she tries to sit next to us. When Dany gets up from the sofa, Frizzy will jump up the sofa and urinate on it.
- when we tell her off she stares us out.
- nevertheless we all like her, she does not have any aggressiveness in her.
- she hates the cold, she sleeps against Dany's belly to keep warm

Jealousy, ailments from grief with diarrhoea and loss of fur suggest Phosphoric acid, which she receives once in a 200K strength.

In a few days all comes back to normal. It takes a little longer for the fur to grow back but that is satisfactory to homeopathic standards. She now also accepts the newly arrived rabbit she previously turned her back on.

Also her attitude of 'reacting' badly when she was reprimanded has disappeared; she is not sensitive to the owner's remarks any more. (Phosphoric acid has the following delusion: thinks that he/she is laughed at)

It is obvious that in this case Phosphoric acid would have helped Frizzy from the beginning. The author comments that he has missed the observation of the owners telling him: 'she acts as if she if she is laughed at'.

The rather aggressive attitude is unusual in this remedy. This should never be a reason not to prescribe a remedy. The absence of a 'typical' characteristic of a remedy or the presence of an unusual observation should never be a reason not to give a remedy if it has been selected using solid homeopathic symptoms. One should never assume that we fully 'know' the picture of a remedy.

14) I am so morally affected that I forget I have a serious problem. (E. De Beukelaer)

Billy was rescued two months ago, he is a gun dog mix; he had a tendency to escape. His new owners had him castrated soon after his arrival to try and curb his escapist behaviour.

When he was first bought into my surgery (by a friend of the owners), the castration wound was very infected and bleeding. This had started a few days after the castration; several treatments tried by the practice that had operated on him had not produced any results.

On examination: Billy has a mild temperature. He was still very lively and eating and drinking normal. Stools were normal. The operation wound is a real mess: there is infected and necrotic tissue everywhere and blood is continually oozing from the wound.

The decision is made to surgically clean the wound and try to stop the bleeding by stitching and cauterization. Billy is also given two types of devices to stop him licking his wound: his owner calls him Houdini for his ability to twist and turn and take off any form of Elizabethan collar or continue to lick his wound while he has the biggest size collar around his neck.

The incessant licking and pulling at the wound is the likely cause of the mess.

The surgery goes well and we manage to stop Billy licking his wound. The infection is soon under control but the bleeding starts again after a few days. Not just a little bleeding; puddles and puddles everywhere!

I find out a little more about him: Billy doesn't like his owners. He still makes efforts to escape. His appetite and endeavour are not affected by the surgery or subsequent blood loss.

Several conventional and homeopathic remedies (Arnica, Phosphorus, Hamamellis, Bellis perennis (i.e. prescription made based on reputed effectiveness)) are given with no result.

It is time to sit down and think really homeopathically: what is the most striking thing in this case?

In spite of the important blood loss, Billy hardly seems to show signs of anemia and continues to display never-ending bouts of energy. He does not seem to care at all about his condition. On the other hand his rescuing and re-homing does not go smoothly, there is no bonding with his owners; usually rescued dogs are really pleased with their arrival into a new family (this is also the reason why there is no further information that could be gathered on the case).

Based on these two observations, Billy is given a dose of Phosphoric acid 30k twice per day. The second day the bleeding stops. The third day the remedy is stopped and a week later the wound in perfectly healed. All the anti-licking devices are taken off him.

A month later the friend of Billy's owner (who has been bringing the dog into the surgery throughout this episode) explains how Billy has made peace with his new family. He is now happily settled.

This is another case of Phosphoric acid apparently contradicting with its usual remedy picture being a remedy for signs of mental and physical 'exhaustion'.

15) My suffering is atrocious! (E. De Beukelaer)

A 4 weeks old calf suffers from typical yellow calf diarrhoea. He has been on antibiotics and re-hydration treatment for two days. His condition does not change. Four other calves that had the same problems are all on the mend with the same treatment.

I ask the farmer what strikes him in the case.

"When we go into his pen he is very frightened and crouches against the back of his pen. He trembles with fear and looks very panicky. Otherwise he stands with his head down and munches some straw without any purpose. We rarely see him lying down. He hardly drinks any water or milk."

I can imagine a calf being afraid of the farmer after having received one or two antibiotic injections but this seems a little over the top. This, alternating with his dull state, is also peculiar.

The following symptoms are used: fear of being approached, dullness during fever, thirstless during diarrhoea.

Three remedies cover these symptoms: Belladonna, Ignatia and Chamomilla.

Chamomilla is selected because of the over-exaggerated reaction of this calf.

One dose in XMK and 12 hours later all is back to normal.

In this case the dilution used was very high. This was because I did not have any other dilution of this remedy with me at the time of the consultation. Generally it is not too much of a problem to use such dilutions in real acute diseases as long as they are not repeated too often. In any case it is more important to use the right remedy than to worry about the right dilution.

One should be very wary of using them for chronic cases because they can really shake up the patient and sometimes cause unnecessary aggravations of unpleasant symptoms to the patient. They can also hide a further aggravation in the patient's health state.

16) Too many pears or lack of attention? (A Duchamps)

This mynah (a black bird with orange streaks on the side that is a good imitator of the human voice) is brought in for 'convulsing'. It started three weeks ago and has been getting worse since. The owners are very worried.

The little bird looks very poorly. His feathers are sticking out in all directions and he trembles all over. The trembling becomes so bad that it looks more like convulsions. The poor bird then loses his balance and falls off his perch.

He often falls off his perch. Once he is on the floor of his cage he hides himself in a box that sits in the bottom. After a while he manages with great difficulty to climb onto his perch again. Soon he starts to tremble again, at first a little, then more and more until he falls off again.

He doesn't eat and talk anymore.

The son says that it is their fault: the family has been very busy in their bakery business and has been feeding him irregularly. Only the youngest son has been giving him pears, which he really likes. As a result his feathering, that normally takes place at this time of the year, has gone off course.

The author dispenses some vitamins and adds a dose of Cuprum in his drinking water without telling the owner about the homeopathic remedy.

When he goes to buy his bread two days later, the baker's wife tells him that within hours the trembling had stopped and the bird started to sing and speak again; she added: "your vitamins are really strong".

The prescription was based on two symptoms: desire to hide and convulsions when eruptions (feathering) don't break out. The author agrees that the choice of the last symptom is very debatable but what counts is the result.

17) Jealousy is really a bad characteristic. (E. De Beukelaer)

This is the story of another bird, a gray parrot this time, called Coco. Parrots typically bond very much with one particular person. This resembles their behaviour in the wild where they live in couples that never separate.

A young man is her proud owner. He just moved in with his pregnant girlfriend; Coco is not impressed at all! She talks much less and when the girlfriend approaches the cage, she shouts and hisses.

Coco is usually very close to her owner. He could hold her and stroke her. This is now only occasionally possible when the girlfriend is not around.

It is when the baby is born that I am called out for advice: Coco had laid an egg and started brooding. When the egg was taken away another egg followed. A third egg followed when the second was taken away and so on until the fifth egg, which was left in the cage. Coco's owner started to worry that she would lose too much energy laying all these eggs because she also ate much less then usual.

This is a typical case of jealousy in parrots.

The following symptoms were used: ailments from jealousy and milk present in non-pregnant women. I agree that the second symptom is a very wide interpretation but it guided me to Phosphorus. (I pinched this idea from a fellow homeopath)

One 30C dose in the drinking water brought everything back to normal. The egg could be taken away and no others followed.

Coco also settled her feud with the girlfriend. She would now accept from time to time to be scratched around the head. She still is very attached to her original owner but that is normal for parrots.

18) I am just a humble worker and it affects my locomotion. (E De Beukelaer)

Chanel is a two year old golden retriever bitch. She is the kindest dog in the world. Sadly, already at this age she shows signs of hip dysplasia and is more or less constantly stiff on her left hind leg. To prevent her from taking painkillers for the rest of her life, it is decided to try and find a suitable homeopathic remedy.

There is not much to say about Chanel: she has all the classical symptoms associated with hip pain and has the usual kind and mild character of her breed. After a long consultation, not much homeopathically useful has come out to distinguish one or another remedy. Chanel likes eating, loves the family, is obedient, never does anything wrong, is friendly to all visitors and family, prefers the fresh air but shies from the sun on a nice day; all the usual things many retrievers do and like.

I then ask her owner what is the most striking feature of Chanel, or the most annoying one. He replies: "She is too obedient. She always has done everything we asked her from the first go." There was a slight tone of annoyance in the client's voice when he made this remark. This was therefore an important remark.

There is a French book (by Guy Loutan, a Swiss homeopath) that sums up themes that are associated with certain remedies. Under the chapter 'obeys too easily' the remedy Formica rufa is mentioned (the ant). I remembered that this remedy has a long list of symptoms associated with rheumatism and that one author accentuated its relationship to the hip joint.

Chanel receives one dose of the remedy in the 200K strength.

I see her a year later for vaccination. There has been no more limping since the remedy and her owner confirmed that she has gained in assurance and character.

19) I have an unusual problem, I need an unusual remedy. (M. Brunson)

Uton is a 5 year old West Highland White terrier. Two weeks ago both of his front legs became paralysed. His hind legs are normal: he uses them to push himself forward, rubbing his chin on the floor. No specific diagnosis has been established for this very unusual infirmity.

The first day he seemed completely lost and became agitated when he tried to get up. There has been no fever. At the same time infected and painful patches have appeared on the skin over his spine and on a few places on his left flank.

Steroids and antibiotics solve the skin problem but not the paralysis.

Uton is then presented to the homeopathic vet.

The owner explains:

"He still eats normally. His thirst has increased since the steroids. When he wants something he barks. He adapts his barking depending on what he wants. He is still happy and wags his tail.

Before he appeared delicate when he was eating. Now it looks as if he has more strength in his jaw.

He is mild, cautious, dynamic, affectionate and intelligent. Very regularly it seems as if he talks to us.
He is stubborn. Some things we have to repeat over and over again. He repeatedly urine marks one corner in the house. When he urinates against a tree he goes around it to make sure his scent is present on all sides. He hates the rain. During the summer he likes the sun. The first day of his illness he was very restless."
Rhus tox 30C one dose.

Two days later, not much change but Uton is brighter and he receives a second dose of Rhus tox 30C.
Another two days later he seems brighter again: Rhus tox 200K. Uton's mobility improves but the front legs stay paralysed.

A new remedy selection is made and Plumbum 200K is administered a week later.
After three more days, still no change in his front legs.
There is a new symptom: "his voice is modified, he barking has become weak." The owner also tells that before he used to lie on his abdomen when he felt too hot.

A new repertorisation is made using paralysis upper limbs (this is uncommon in dogs), skin eruption suppurating, skin eruption painful and voice weak.
This produces 16 remedies. The author eliminates one after another because they don't seem to fit the case. There is one remedy out of the sixteen that attracts his attention: Baryta sulf.
Baryta carbonicum is known for its paralysis of the upper limbs and Sulphur fits some aspects of his behaviour. The combination of the two under the form of Baryta sulf seems interesting. (The author explains he has no experience or particular knowledge of this remedy).
Baryta sulf 200K once. Over the next days Uton regains the activity of his front limbs. After ten days he is still very weak on them and the progress is stagnating. A further 200K dose and he recuperates completely from his illness.

135

There is not much comment to make on this remedy that is not especially well known. The case is a further example that all efforts must be made to base a prescription on what the patient 'tells' us. Homeopathy answers to the patient and not to set rules. The case also shows how useful it is to persist in searching for the appropriate remedy. In many occasions after some time a new symptom or observation helps in finding a more appropriate remedy.

20) I cannot cope with emotions but I still feel strong. (A Duport)

Hunter is a German shepherd. He is two years old and has recurrent attacks of piroplasmosis (a blood parasite transmitted by ticks). He has been treated conventionally for this affliction for some time now.

When he is presented to the homeopathic vet, he hasn't eaten for 10 days. Nevertheless as soon as he gets some attention he displays his usual energy.

Spontaneously, his owner tells his story:

"He was born the 5th of January in a reputable breeding kennel. I chose him when he was 6 weeks old because after having played for an hour with his brothers and sisters he came to me and put his paw on my knees.

Very soon he has filled in the gap that was left when our previous dog died. He was very well in himself; very balanced, happy, kind, affectionate, sociable and very easy to train. He is a playful dog and as a young puppy developed the habit of keeping his toys tidily in his bed and putting them back there as soon as he finished playing with them.

He was not a destructive puppy; he has just slightly nibbled one of the chairs. He adapts very easily and loves playing and running. He loves the car and started to defend the car before he defended the house.

Although he is a very active dog, he does not wake up very early and does not want to be woken up before his hour.

He is very sensitive towards us; he senses the least tension, drop in attention or change in habits. It affects him tenfold; he sees it as a slander towards him.

He goes everywhere with us, he is seldom alone; he hates being on his own. When we leave him alone he waits on his bed until we are back and then we receive a very exuberant greeting.

He is very good with other animals. He has a dwarf rabbit as a friend and plays gently with him. He likes cats (they don't like him) and small dogs. It is a little more difficult with bigger dogs. In the beginning, he takes a defensive attitude. After a while he accepts play with them and there will be no problem.

On a few occasions there were fights; they stopped early enough to prevent any damage.

Anything dressed in feathers is at risk with him. There are very few birds in our garden because of him.

He is a good guard dog but shows no aggression towards people. He prefers ladies to men and loves children; the younger the better.

The only place where nobody apart from his family can touch him is when he is in the car.

He has great patience with an adolescent handicapped child in the family.

He is not excessively jealous, when he is affected this reflects in his health, not in his behaviour towards the other animals.

From the age of four months he became difficult to feed; he eats little for a dog of his size. He refuses to eat the same food twice. He does not tolerate tinned food very well, he prefers dry food but the biscuits have to be small. He likes fresh table scraps as long as they are not too fat but doesn't eat vegetables and fruit. He used to love raw eggs but has refused to eat eggs over the last few weeks, especially when they were cooked. He also likes milk (drinks a bowl every day) and dainties as long as they are not too sweet. He takes medicines as if they are sweets but doesn't like chocolate.

He only eats well when he really likes something, for a while this has been tinned cat food based on fish. If we overfill his dish his appetite goes away immediately. He loses his weight very quickly during the periods of low appetite.

He had his first attack of piroplasmosis when he was six months old; this showed by a lack of fitness and a diminished desire to play. (Usually this disease causes very high fever, blood in the urine and considerable lethargy.) Since then these episodes have occurred frequently and have been treated conventionally.

He has a tendency to eczema on the base of his tail and on the side of his hind legs. When he was young he often had weeping eyes. We suspect this was related to the feeding of tins because when we stopped the tins it disappeared altogether. He frequently comes home with ticks and fleas.

When he was one year old, a brown patch developed on the inside of both ears. He has a tendency to be constipated. His diet does not seem to have any influence on this. Only a top quality brand of dry food improved it somewhat.

There are some unspecific irregularities in his blood results. Every time he receives one of these injections for his disease, he develops a large engorged swelling on the site of injection that takes weeks to disappear. He tends to 'react' to the medicines that are given for his eczema lesions.

My previous dog had a very strong and proud character; he never gave in regardless of his painful hip condition. Hunter is the contrary; the least problem makes him depressive. He then stays in the house with me and looks at me as if I am the cause of his suffering. He never gets tired of being hugged, petted and kissed by his 'family'. Apart from young children he does not look for affection from strangers.

It seems that each period of illness is caused by a small change in our attention towards him.

This time his illness started when we kept our parents' dog. He was very upset by this presence."

Based on ailments from grief, refuses to eat and playful, Hyosciamus 30C one dose is given. He improves the next day and eats better for fourteen days. He then becomes more 'difficult' in his behaviour.
This is an indicator that the remedy was not homeopathic.

Three weeks later he is down again. He refuses any food apart from milk and looks for cool places. He prefers the car to any other place.

Eat refuses to, ailments from grief and milk desire, orientates the homeopath to Phosphoric acid; one 30C dose.

"Returning home from the surgery Hunter vomited several times and was very weak for 24 hrs. He then picked up and started eating again. The fourth day after a long walk with my husband, suddenly his eyes brightened up and the next day he was back in full shape. Since then, he has become the dog we knew before."

Hunter returns to the surgery 5 months later; he is down again. "Again he has this interrogating look and isolates himself. He seems to have a weakness in his hind legs. His appetite is still fine but he refuses his milk in the morning.

Something has changed in our family; my husband has opened a new shop and has rarely been at home for a few weeks. I also am absent more than usual. Therefore Hunter frequently stays on his own which he hates. He never shows us his worries when we come back; we always receive a happy welcome.

He doesn't want to play for the moment and goes to lay on my bed which he usually only does when he is on his own. What is new is that he has these sudden erections and start to imitate a coition, which is followed by the emission of some fluid. He seems surprised when this happens and it upsets him. If we start to play ball with him it all disappears quickly.

He must feel some uneasiness because he chews his feet and the places where he used to develop his eczema."

A dose of Phosphoric acid 30C solves the case. In 36 hrs Hunter is back to his usual self, apart from maybe an increased demand for fussing.

Last news from Hunter was two years later when he was still doing very well since the last dose of medicine.

21) Hell breaks loose in the consult room. (B. Heude)

This is a story about a case of kennel cough, an infectious disease in dogs which is reputed to be difficult to treat.

The client has a small breeding holding with a variety of breeds living peacefully together. The people are very good with their animals and there is a nice atmosphere in the big dog family. They don't vaccinate against kennel cough.

After a weekend at a dog show, 5 dogs start to cough on the way home.

" They cough when they get excited; they cough when we come home and when we leave. They never cough when they run or play. Rouza has a little cough when she rises. Isthar tries to expectorate something when she coughs. Iron has a dry cough, often two attacks, followed by a fruitless effort to vomit. Fred has a dry cough, mostly two or three attacks. He also has swollen tonsils"

Nervous cough, cough two or three attacks, swollen tonsils indicate phosphorus. A 30K dose twice per day for four days.

Two dogs get better in one day and two take four days before the cough disappears. A few other dogs that develop the disease from contact with them also get better quite rapidly with the remedy.

The case is not an example of spectacular homeopathic activity but the result can be judged satisfying, no antibiotics have been used and none of the patients have become chronic coughers, which happens frequently.

The owners don't follow up the recommendations of their vet and neglect to prevent contact between the coughing dogs and the rest of the pack. The disease is allowed to spread but it happens quietly.

For more then a month all seems fine. Then suddenly a litter of 7 week old Staffordshire pups start to cough.

When they are brought to the surgery, they 'invade' the consultation room, piddle and poo everywhere and attack all the chairs and the table. They have a loose cough, six or more attacks, which doesn't stop their hooligan behaviour for a second.

"They were vaccinated by your colleague four days ago. The coughing started one evening, two days ago, when there was a cold northeastern wind. They continue to scoff down their food. None of them has a temperature. When they cough they make a snoring noise, they sound engorged. We wormed them yesterday, they were full of worms."

It is tempting to use the same remedy that produced good results on the previous expression of kennel cough. This outbreak can be regarded as being very closely related to the one that happened the month before; there has been no exchanges with dogs from outside the kennels. For completeness the author decides to make a new repertorisation to give the pups the best possible chance.

Cough wind (east and north), vaccinations after, worms, rattling cough. Sepia is best represented and given in 30C dilution twice in 12 hours.

Followed a noticeable aggravation of the cough for a few hours. The next day they were all fine except for one pup that continued to cough for a week.

One more example to show that it is possible to treat pure infectious diseases without the need for antibiotics. When groups are treated it is common to have a small percentage of individuals that doesn't respond to the remedy.

22) I have fear when I decide it. (JP Spillbauer)

Praline is a 15 year old mare who has been suffering from chronic emphysema for many years.

Every summer she has conjunctivitis, nasal discharge and facial inflammation; in the winter she starts to cough and develops respiratory distress. She cannot be ridden anymore because of her breathing problems.

"A few years ago she had a few bouts of colic and caught several colds. Two years before the respiratory problems started the osteopath 'unblocked' several things. The allergy started after the owners and horse moved a few years ago. She only had one episode then. She regularly suffers from mud-rash."

"She has lost a lot of weight since her emphysema. We have wormed her several times. She hangs out at the bottom of the field. She stands there staring. When she sees us; she calls us. She is in 'love' with the pony we bought after we moved.

Before he arrived, it was nearly impossible to load her in the van. Now she follows the pony without hesitating. As soon as they were together he tried to drink from her, she kicked him off. From the next day they were best friends.

We can catch her easily. This wasn't the case before. She is anxious but not nasty. She doesn't stand up to other horses. She can be scared by a sign on the road. Sometimes she panics; it is incredible: as if an insect stings her. It lasts for a minute. She calms when I get angry with her. When she panics like this, she walks all over us and cannot be reasoned with mildness, I have to get cross. She can have her head covered with flies without being worried!

She doesn't like to jump. Even a one-foot jump she would refuse. She has never been an adept of working.

An equine dentist once commented: "she likes to understand what you do to her". Strangely enough, the osteopath had made exactly the same remark a few months before.

She makes me think of a cat; she will come to us if she decides to. She wants tranquillity. When she didn't want to go into the lorry she didn't go in but she was never violent. When she says no that means no! To give her a worming dose it is a big affair, it is not possible to do this in a hurry; she needs time to accept the tube in her mouth.

She had a foal when she was three; it was an accident, just like her; she is also born to an unknown father.

Our neighbour told us she is very sensitive to our absences; she seems anxious in the field. We cannot say that she is affectionate."

The homeopath uses the following symptoms: delusion sees insects, fear of jumping, fear of being touched.

This orientates to Belladonna, Tarentula, Hyosciamus and Stramonium.

Belladonna is administrated because this remedy seemed most appropriate; Belladonna lives by its own rules and doesn't learn; one has to re-explain things over and over again.

Belladonna is also known for its efficiency in lung problems. Using the renowned activity knowledge about a remedy may be helpful in distinguishing between several remedies that seem indicated in a case.

One dose in 200K strength.
Nothing seems to happen but her usual complaints don't reappear. Eight months later, during the winter, there is a mild re-occurrence of respiratory symptoms very quickly stopped by a further dose of Belladonna 30K.

Two years later she is still fine and can be ridden again regularly without problems.

Belladonna is a reputed remedy for fever but in the hands of an experienced homeopath can solve many situations.

23) Not a silver bullet but a silver pill (E. De Beukelaer)

Jilly is a 13-year-old female spaniel who enjoyed an active life with daily exercise until she is brought to the surgery on a Sunday. She has been unable to get up since the previous evening. She yelps from pain when moved or touched around the back. Her temperature is 41.5° C.
My colleague hospitalises the patient. She receives anti-inflammatory and antibiotic treatment.
No improvement on Monday. X-rays show extensive spondylitis all along the spine from thoracic to spinal vertebrae.
Treatment is pursued with no further result. On Tuesday the patient still cannot lift her head and temperature levels out at 41° C.

I examine the patient on Tuesday and notice the following: sensitivity in the legs is conserved, pupils are unequal, the patient is aware of her surroundings, she can hardly lift her head, the spine is very painful, she feels very hot.

The owner is very concerned about the quality of life for Jilly and euthanasia is considered. I ask, and obtain, 24 hours delays to see whether homeopathy can make a difference.

I retain the following symptoms:
Pupils unequal.
Hectic fever.
Sudden appearance of illness.
Weakness from pain.
Two remedies attract attention: Belladonna and Argentum metallicum. The second, remedy is ordered to arrive the next day.

Because of the likelihood of some efficacy, Belladonna (which was available) is administered in 30K dilution once every hour 5 times. All conventional treatment was stopped on Tuesday morning.

The next morning the temperature has come down to 39.0° C and Jilly can lift her head. She doesn't mind being touched and transported any more.

The improvement was satisfying but seemed not fully homeopathic. The second remedy arrived on Wednesday and was given twice in the morning. Twitching of the neck muscles and a return of the weakness followed. By 4 pm she stood up in her cage by herself. The next day she could walk again and started eating and drinking. She went home on Friday, without any further treatment.

A week later on Saturday, Jilly was seen again because she found it difficult to get up. Argentum metallicum was administered, followed by rapid improvement. Two weeks later she was running her usual walks again.

Jilly is fine for two months, when she relapses and is put to sleep in my absence.

In this case it was unfortunate that I did not insist sufficiently for the owner to come back to have a follow up consultation. Further administrations of the remedy may have prevented such an early relapse.

It is interesting to see how Belladonna was effective but not fully homeopathic. This is a nice example of how remedies can be partially effective without having a profound homeopathic activity that warrants such better quality improvements.

24) Coldness from sunstroke. (S. Crouzet)

Galupka is a pure Arab mare who had her first foal at 3.5 years old following a 'mishap' in the field; nature is sometimes difficult to stop when it wants to preserve its continuity, especially in the still pristine countryside where Galupka lives.

The first few days after the foaling all goes well.

It is the middle of the summer and the sun is burning high up in the sky when she is found, at 3 pm lying down in the field. She needs firm encouragement to get up and walk to the stables. She lies down as soon as she arrives there.

Her legs are cold, she sweats all over, her respiration is laboured, heart rate is low, she is anxious and agitated and her legs spread out with a certain rigidity. (diagnosis: hypocalcaemia or eclampsia).

There is only 1/8th of the normal amount available of calcium necessary for a horse. A drip is set up (with difficulty). Somebody is sent out to collect extra calcium bags from the closest vets practice many miles away. The owner of the horse who uses homeopathic remedies herself administrates Camphora XM. The mare's state becomes worse.

Awaiting the arrival of more calcium, something needs to be done; her heart rate goes down and she goes into ophistotonus (head turned backwards).

The homeopathic vet who is only on holiday has none of his books with him but recalls Carbo vegetabilis as a remedy indicated in desperate cases with sweating and respiratory difficulties and administrates a few drops of the XM strength.

Twenty minutes later the mare is up and eating hay. She receives the rest of her calcium dose two hours later.

From there all goes well.

This is one of the many cases where in desperate situations the right homeopathic remedy can be life saving. Also, and many homeopaths will admit this, luck in finding or deciding on the right remedy is always an appreciable help. The right attitude can increase the chance of benefiting from some extra luck.

25) Charlie the protecting 'father'. (JP Spillbauer)

Charlie suffers with chronic infectious dermatitis of the ventral part of his body from head to tail. He is a 2 year old German Shepherd dog. He has been treated for a long time with conventional medicines.

"He was one month old when we had him. Two other pups from his litter we see regularly also have skin problems, just like their mother. When she had her puppies she was tired. Her owners sold the puppies early because the bitch lacked milk.

Charlie is a nice, gentle and playful dog. He is very good with our other dog, a poodle, which tries to dominate him. When it goes too far Charlie just stops him.

Charlie is like a father to the poodle; as soon as he runs too much, Charlie stops him. If he goes out too far, Charlie brings him back. It is the same with us; if we go too far away, Charlie takes us by the arm and brings us close by.

He seems bored. He is alone during the day. It is better since our son comes home during lunch hour. When I take the poodle with me to work Charlie is not jealous at all. He is tranquil.

He loves children. He doesn't like loud noises or when there is too much activity in our house. Generally he is playful and happy. His skin problems don't seem related to anything at all."

Question from the vet: why did you say 'he is like a father to the poodle?'

" That is really him; if my son wants to ride his go-cart, Charlie stops him from doing so and bites the wheels. He doesn't want him to go on it. It has always been like this. I have the impression that he is trying to protect us from getting hurt.

146

When we play fight with our son, he intervenes to stop it. He has no aggressiveness whatsoever; he comes up to us and whines in the hope that we stop. He always seem to prevent us from being hurt although nothing has ever happened to us."

In the consulting room, Charlie has a sniff around and seems uneasy.

"He wants us to open the door so he can leave. He is very patient, he was easy to educate. He adapts very easily everywhere.

He protects us but he is no guard dog. He doesn't stop people from entering the house but people are afraid of him.

Even when the skin is at its worse, he is quite well. The weather has no influence on him. Once when we went to the sea with him, his coat became shiny again. He loves swimming."

The author is surprised by the emphasis on the fatherly character by his owners.

In the thematic repertory (G Loutan) under father figure comes Arnica as a remedy.

One MK dose and all his skin problems disappear. He is seen again seven months later. He only needed a mild cleansing of his ears. The skin is perfect and shining.

Arnica, remedy for bruises? There is more to homeopathy! Also remember that in an earlier case there was a cat that protected the other kitten in the house but the remedy that worked was different; one symptom is not enough to decide on an appropriate remedy.

26) Little by little they tell us their story and we find their remedy. (A Duport)

More skin problems. This six year old pointer bitch is presented for eruptions on the side of the left hind leg. They started 15 days ago. The owner is worried that they may get infected when she goes running in the countryside.

There are several circular, suppurating, slightly bleeding patches the size of a pea grouped in a surface the size of a large coin. There is no itch.

"She lives outside in kennels together with a few other working dogs. She is an excellent gun dog and works every day. She has always been healthy since she was bought at the age of four months. She is not bothered by the weather. She is only interested in working.

She is a nervous dog, always active. The restlessness is increased when she is on heat. On the moment she is a little over the top. She is very attached to my husband but completely indifferent to me."

A rapid prescription of Graphites 30C (twice per day 3 days), based on the aspect of the lesion, improves the skin within a week.

Five months later: Reappearance of the same skin problem. This time the aspect is dry. She is still very nervous and agitated. She works really well; "she is a pleasure to have.

She drinks often in small quantities. It seems that on wet days she has less energy. She does not like the heat very much. She is not happy when we touch the lesion."

Although the vet has some doubts about the remedy, because of the previous success, Graphites 30C is given again twice per day three days.
Again, the lesion disappears within the week.

Ten months later: She has lost weight and her appetite has increased. She steals the other dogs' food. This is a sign that the remedy was not homeopathic to the dog; the skin problems have been suppressed and the patient is getting worse in herself.

"We have been away for a week. She stayed in the kennel during that time. It seems that she has suffered from this She hasn't been on heat; normally she is very regular.

She is not an anxious dog."

The author comments that he has made a bad repertorisation this time; based on the following symptoms: emaciation with ravenous appetite, suppressed eruptions, forsaken feeling. Calcarea carb makes no difference.

Two weeks later, she continues to lose weight and develops a superficial staphylococcus infection on the front legs.
Graphites is used again to no effect.

Three weeks later, skin lesions develop over all the joints. They are wet, yellow, mildly hemorrhagic and itchy. She is so hungry she started to eat her faeces. She still loses weight and has developed several bald batches.
She has still the same character. Temperature is increased and she still hasn't come on heat.
Based on the appetite and weight loss, Iodum 30C is administered to no effect.

One month later, she becomes sad and loses her dynamism. "She always want to be with us, especially with the husband. She whines from the least upset. To go to the toilet she always goes away, far away."
This time, the author commented, he has a good look at his file and selects the following symptoms: emaciation and increased appetite, weeps about trifles, hides to go to the toilet.
The obvious remedy is Natrum muriaticum XM one dose. (the 'close' relationship with the husband is very indicative for this remedy)
There is an immediate result. Three days later she has gained 700 grams, she seems happy and she has come on heat.

Ten days later his colleague consults the dog. In ten days a mammary tumour has developed. It is decided to operate on the spot.
All goes well, she comes back on heat two months later and the skin is beautiful.

Two months later, another heat appears. She also needs a cleansing treatment for her ears. Skin, weight and behaviour are fine.

One month later, a new tumour appears in no time.

She receives a new dose of Natrum muriaticum XM. The tumour stops growing and disappears two months later. (Confirmed by the conventional colleague).

One year later she suddenly starts lose weight again, like she is melting away. Appetite and thirst are normal. She is sad but she still plays with the other dog. She has very discreet heat symptoms.

Ten days prior, her owner had gone to hospital for hip replacement.

Natrum mur. 30C.

Two days later; disaster; she is dying. She seems to have given up. She is put on a drip and Natrum muriaticum XM is administered. She recovers in a few days.

She is back her usual self over the next year until she is left alone again for a short while. Same scenario, same remedy, same dilution and a few days later all is well again.

Eight months later she is brought in with a stomach torsion. Emergency operation and one dose on Natrum mur. XM but she doesn't make it and dies a few hours later.

Afterwards the owner mentioned how good she has been the last few months. She had now moved into the house because the other dog had died. She had never been so happy in her life.

The author commented that is was possible to find Natrum muriaticum from the first consultation (with hindsight this is often possible in homeopathic cases but doesn't indicate any incompetence, it is due to the nature of homeopathic medicine). In this case he considers that Ebene died in full health from the consequences of an 'accident'. He cannot explain why he gave the 30C dose when Ebene came in ill again and considers this to be the cause of the sudden aggravation.

It is possible to debate on how perfect the remedy was in this case. The remedy has certainly offered a good quality last few years to this bitch, but there are two observations that can throw a shade on the 'homeopathicity' of the prescription in this case. First she develops a tumour after the first dose of Nat-m, secondly she is very much aggravated when she receives a 30C dose. The stomach torsion, interpreted by the author as an accident may give rise to doubts as to the quality of the health balance acquired after having received several doses of the medicine. The use of very high dilutions (in this case XMK) can make things difficult to interpret; very high dilutions may have such a profound effect on patients that they can keep them going without resulting in a cure. This comment can be seen as hairsplitting, certainly when the patient has benefited so well, but it is important to make such considerations to allow for continuous improvement in homeopathic prescription and excelling in prescription for the benefit of the patient.

But even when the remedy is not perfectly homeopathic, patients can still find great benefit.

27) Tell me how you wee and I will find your remedy. (P Froment)

This is the story of Fido who is a large longhaired dog of unidentifiable origin. He arrived at his owner's house when he was young. He is extremely kind but very cautious.

He needs some time to accept strangers but after a while he is very cuddly. He was 'hit' when he was young and still had a deformed vertebra since this accident.

He has difficulties urinating and is constipated. The diagnosis is inflammation of the prostate. There is not much homeopathic to go on. That is why he receives a hormone injection and a liver tonic.

When he relapses three weeks later it is obvious that help from homeopathy is very advisable.

The vet asks: 'is there anything particular you noted about him?'

"He cannot urinate while standing but when he lies down urine will dribble unnoticed. When he sleeps, his left hind leg keeps on moving laterally from left to right. His head is trembling, there are spasms that go from his right lip to his right ear"

In the repertory the following symptoms are found: he cannot urinate while standing but lying down he urinates a few drops, cannot urinate standing but urine flows when sitting down, motions of the extremities during sleep, tics of the right side of the head while sleeping, tics of the right side of the face.

Causticum is present in all these rubrics.

One 200K dose is given and he is well from the next day.

He needs a second dose (MK) six months later for a reoccurrence.

Two years later his is still fine and has a slightly enlarged prostate. There has been no further necessity for treatment.

28) 'I need some petrol to restart'. (L. Guiouillier)

Nocturne is a Normandy milking cow that has been troubled by a host of different ailments over the last months.

The farmer describes her as follows:

"She was anxious and agitated when she needed to be inseminated. It has taken three cycles before she became pregnant. When she calved, another cow took away her calf; she searched for it all day to find it in the evening. (Note: this is very unusual) In the milking parlour she was very nervous; she trembled from fear, she is very sensitive but she never tried to kick us. She calmed down after a few months. She has never had mastitis.

It took many artificial inseminations before she got in calf again. Her troubles begin after her second calving.

Her problems started with an infection of the foot, treated conventionally, from which she didn't recover completely. She limps, loses appetite and fifteen days later an abscess broke open on the edge of the claws.

A month later she started to cough and developed a fever. This episode is treated with antibiotics. Fourteen days later she developed mastitis. Her udder is warm, painful, hard and she kicks when touched. There is a quick improvement with antibiotics.

She then develops ringworm lesions on the head, neck and hindquarters.

She is quiet and seems sad and anxious. She doesn't like to be approached but accepts catching. There is a yellow discharge from the left nostril."

She receives Cuprum 30C.

This remedy did not have the desired effect because 14 days later she develops a very severe form of mastitis. When she walks around in the herd, she lifts her head; the farmer says: "it is as if she is asking for help". He also reminds the vet about her previous wild character.

'Helplessness' and 'wildness' point towards several remedies. Phosphorus 9C is administered twice per day for three days.

She improves but after five days the cure is not complete.

A new repertorisation based on wildness, helpless, fear approached, weakness during fever and unhealthy skin.

From the remedy list, Petroleum is selected. Two 15C doses at eight days interval.

Rapidly her udder returns to normal and she finds serenity again. Her fearful behaviour never comes back. The health of her udder is closely monitored for seven months with excellent marks.

29) 'I am affectionate and independent'. (D Notre-Dame)

For Izzy, coming on heat means a period of lack of appetite and lethargy. Being a four year old Rough collie she should be full of energy all the time.

The first week of this period she is very agitated, then she becomes lethargic which can last up to two months.

"She has a very delicate digestive system. At the least upset she has blood in her stools. Her stools are usually pale and she produces them accompanied by much flatulence. She comes on heat every nine months. Before each period she refuses to be stroked and walks away.

She is introverted; she doesn't show her feelings. She is easy-going and very sensitive. She loves everybody except cats and anything that attacks her. She doesn't defend herself against people; she goes away if they hurt her.

She will eat anything but especially craves fish.

She is sensitive to noise, especially noises from engines; she attacks them. She will be frightened by a falling lid.

She hates any differences of opinion and her mistress' 'anger' attacks. She also hates thunder and, when she was young, the wind.

She stays alone no problems, she is affectionate but independent. She loves fish."

On examination she has a sensitive liver and there is a patch of regressing eczema on the left shoulder.

The following symptoms are used: weakness during menses, weakness after menses, clear stools, fish desire, menses late, fear of thunderstorm, introspection, sensitive to noise.

Phosphorus is administered in 200K strength; no result.

Two weeks later, Sepia 9C (which came second in the repertorisation) one dose and she finds her energy again. Her owner comments that she is back to what she was when she was young.

This is a nice sepia case: 'I like you but not too close'.

30) But I like it when I exercise! (E De Beukelaer)

Tina is a 20 year old very small pony of unknown origin.

During the winter of 1999-2000, she lost her appetite, became 'sad', made small faecal balls, coughed a little and lost weight. Blood samples suggested some unspecified liver complaint. After worm and liver treatment, she picked up in the spring, when the grass was growing.

The following year, the cough reappeared in the autumn. She lost appetite again, the faecal balls became small again and the sadness also came back.

The homeopathic consultation takes place in April 2001; she is still not doing well.

"She had one foal ten years ago. It was very difficult to make her accept the stallion. She looked after her foal normally. She has a lot of character, she is obstinate."

Her respiration is laboured and auscultation reveals a lot of cracking sounds all over the pulmonary field.

The diagnosis is Chronic Obstructive Pulmonary Disease: not a good prognosis.

"She is better, mentally and respiratorily, when she 'works' at the pony club although she lacks in general condition. I'd like her to be better again because she is brilliant pulling the little cart we have. She will always be in the back of her box or separated from the other ponies when on pasture. When the others come too close to her she will chase them away. Anyway, they all respect her and leave her alone."

The following symptoms are used: Cough in cold wet air, thirstless, ameliorated by physical exertion, aversion to company, and stools like sheep droppings.

Sepia is given for three consecutive days in the 9C Potency. This is followed by a rapid improvement in all the patient's symptoms. She gains her normal weight, is happy again and has a good summer season working at the pony club.

Next winter (2001-2) coughing started again and one dose of Sepia 9C stopped it very quickly. She is still fine (06 2003)

31) A thirsty carpet. (J P Spillbauer)

Zerbino is a fox terrier (13 years old) brought in for excessive drinking.

"He drinks anything he can find. It is an obsession. This has been going for over a year now. He drinks the water in the puddles, the gutter, when it rains and even his own urine. He even doesn't think about urinating anymore.

Sometimes he is fine and calm. Then, suddenly he becomes stressed.

Before, when he was stressed he started to scratch. He had eczema; it has disappeared since he started drinking.

Many veterinarians have been consulted. The end conclusion is always pituitary problems.

It is my husband's dog. I have been with him (husband) for seven years. He works from home. Zerbino usually lies at his feet.

He became ill when we took him with us when we were shooting a film. On this occasion he received less attention. He never stopped following his master.

Before every upset, he developed eczema. Now the eczema has gone and he drinks."

Vet; 'what sort of upset?'

Answer: "don't know"

"He has no sexual activity, although he fights with a few other male dogs. He was a killer; we had several problems because of him. When he doesn't know people he growls. He doesn't like new things but he is not a guard dog. He frightens new people.

When he knows people he is very affectionate. He is always adorable with us, he is calm and never barks.

Sometimes, things get hysterical: he defies me: 'if you don't give me anything to drink I will urinate'. The more he drinks the more he urinates. Sometimes, if I stop him from drinking; he calms down, it is weird."

Vet: ' Why have you called him Zerbino?'

"It means floor-mat in Italian. An Italian gave the name to him because he used to sleep on his belly with his four legs spread out. This habit lasted ten years.

I bought him in a bar; he was the smallest of the litter and had been ill. He caught up later.

The drinking started when we were away filming and he had developed the most impressive eczema again. He stayed by the radiator all the time and cried. The local vet came and gave him a shot of steroids. He stopped scratching and started to drink soon after."

During the whole of the consultation, Zerbino sat in front of the door, away from the people in the consult room but kept an eye on them, without moving but not indifferent.

"Everything he does, he does for ages"

Vet: 'Does he like to stay at home?'

"That must be his problem: he wants to be with us wherever he goes but he would prefer to be home.

Sometimes he can stay in the car for hours without demanding anything to drink."

Eruptions suppressed, sleeps on abdomen, perseverance, desire to go home indicate Bryonia. (note that the drinking symptom was not used to select the remedy)

One 200K dose.

Twelve days later he started to scratch himself. This stopped after a few days and he reduced his drinking habit. A month later all is back to normal. He is more at peace with himself.

Zerbino dies two and a half years later at the age of 16. He never needed any more medication.

32) I am very confident my homeopath will sort me out. (M Brunson)

Not all cases are solved in one or two attempts. A little perseverance helps in these cases, even when thing become desperate.

When Becky was first brought to the surgery, she was two months old. She is a boxer and was bought a week earlier. Only skin and bones are left.

Soon after her arrival she developed loose stools and vomited some red faecal matter containing worms. She doesn't drink or eat and after a few days her urine turns yellow and later green. She sleeps all the time and prefers to stay close to her owners. She still wags her tail when their grandchild comes in.

She wants to lie in the shade, she flees the sun, she doesn't want to be covered and pushes off all covers.

She looks sad but is not weak considering the state she is in.

That is all there is to find a remedy.
Absence of weakness during diarrhoea, urine greenish, thirstless, warmth aggravates, worms, indicate Sulfur.
A 12K dose is given three times per day.

The next day she seems brighter, she ate a small amount of ham (after 4 days of refusing all food) she drinks again.
Sulfur 12K, three times.

The next days she really starts to eat and played with the grandson.
Sulfur 30K once per day. 3 days.

Five days later she is worse again. "She stopped drinking, she is always on our laps, no fever, no interest in anything."

On the symptoms: thirstless, desire to be carried, sad, Pulsatilla 12C three times per day is administered.

No change the next day: stools are yellow, clay like. "She always wants to be in our arms or on our laps. She looks for warmth, she breathes slowly".

Conclusion: wrong remedy. The other remedy that also likes to stay in contact is Phosphorus.

A 12C dilution is administered three times per day.

The next day there is a mild improvement. She has eaten a little. She still stays the whole day on her owner's lap.

Phosphorus 12K three times during the day.

Two days later. No real change.

She hides herself in the consult room. She becomes hypothermic. She hides her head under the covers.

On the symptoms: desire to hide, desire to be carried and anxiety alone, Arsenicum album 12K is given three times during the day.

The next day she is transformed. She eats and she started to follow the other dogs again.

Arsenicum album 30K twice per day during two more days, all problems disappear and Becky picks life up again where it nearly stopped.

There are many cases like this. They often don't get published because the authors are not proud of their successes. In other cases, the homeopath did not get enough chance to arrive at the desired results.

33) How homeopathy brings peace. (M Brunson)

One late afternoon, a client requests a home visit for her elderly poodle. For a few months her poodle bitch has been treated for heart failure and this evening she is really very bad.

She has received diuretics and digitalis drops over the past few months; a conventional colleague looked after her health.

Her respiration is very accelerated, her pulse is slow, she coughs all the time, keeps her head up in the air in an effort to catch for air. She is in a poor condition: when she coughs, her front legs give away and she sometimes loses consciousness during her coughing efforts. She coughs at the least movement she makes. She cannot settle and goes from one place to another. This started a week ago.

She still appreciates being stroked by the vet. Based on the severity of the case and the necessity to move about all the time regardless of exhaustion and the appreciation of being cared for, Arsenicum album 12K is prescribed to be given 5 times in the next 12 hours.

As agreed, the next morning the owner rings the vet with an update, she is in tears but at the same time explains her gratitude and thanks the vet. These are the word she used: "After the first administration of the remedy, she became much calmer. She managed to settle down to sleep. The anxiety in her expression had disappeared. She received a second dose one and a half hours later and then I went upstairs to bed, she followed me and peacefully cuddled up against my back. She hadn't done this for many days; she had been so restless, up and down all the time. Two hours later I woke up to give her the third dose. She was still lying against my back but had died. It was such a nice death, she was so tranquil; it was incredible. I am so happy she died in such a nice way"

This is an other proof of how homeopathy can be of great benefit in a variety of different scenarios.

34) Bold and unreliable. (P Rouchossé)

Elsa is a big Pyrenean sheep dog. She is two years old and has lost all her fur on her abdomen and between her legs. A very thinned-out coat covers the rest of the body. She is very fat and her skin is thin suggesting the likelihood of a hormonal problem. The conventional vet proposes to spay the bitch.

The owners prefer to find a different solution and consult the homeopathic vet.

"She hides herself under the bed as soon as we come home. If we call her she comes and lies close to us and doesn't move at all.

She has suckled a cloth since we have had her (from the age of six months). Her mother died giving birth. Elsa destroys all cardboard boxes she can find when she is alone, especially at night. She always follows Jerry, she has her nose in his hand when they go for a walk, she doesn't leave him for a second. She is very obedient, especially to him.

She is always looking for affection. She is jealous. She puts herself between us, she is jealous of Laura (daughter).

In unknown places she pants, pulls on the lead and coughs.

When Laura prepares her food, she doesn't eat until Jerry is back. She is not really interested in other dogs. When she is on heat she is terrible; she needs constant fussing and she cries all the time. After every heat period she has a phantom pregnancy.

She is a good guard dog; nobody can get into the car, even people she knows. She will bite.

She doesn't like children, she growls and jumps to frighten them.

She drinks small amounts and she doesn't like peas. She will have cherries when we have them. She often vomits yellow bile. She frequently has diarrhoea, very liquid, dark brown. She always has parasites, even if we treat her she still has them.

She first started losing her fur when she was 6-7 months old. When she lost her fur the second time, all her hair fell out in three days.

She loves being outside. As soon as she is sad, she comes up to Jerry and looks at him. She will fall asleep when he strokes her.

She has a fear of water, we cannot wash her, she never comes near water. In the car she sits in a small corner behind Jerry's seat.

She steals, whatever she can find. She has fear of all noises and in the lift.

The worst thing that can happen to her is to say; I don't want to see you any more or to lock her away in a room on her own.

She once stole Laura's teddy. She always has a toy in her mouth. When Jerry is not there she doesn't eat."

Based on the symptoms; ailments from jealousy, fear of water, refuses to eat, weeping during menses, desire company, Hyosciamus 12C is given, one dose.

Three weeks later.

"She is doing very well, she doesn't weep any more, she doesn't hide anymore, she eats well, she wants to play. Her hair hasn't grown back yet"

One week later the fur starts to grow back (and she starts to scratch herself).
Two months later, all the fur has grown back and she is behaving very well.

Three months later, the fur starts to fall out again; another dose of the remedy in 30C and the fur starts to grow again two weeks later.

The local veterinary school diagnoses a hypersensitivity to sexual hormones. No treatment is needed because she is doing very well.

35) Even when I was taken out of my prison, I still lived in a prison. (M Brunson)

Diane is a Labrador bitch who was adopted when she was seven years old. Her new owner had noticed during her walks that Diana lived in a kennel at the rear of a garden. Because she thought this wasn't a life for such a nice dog, she asked her owners whether she could take her on. They 'gladly' parted with their dog.

A few weeks before the homeopathic consultation, she had been treated conventionally (drops etc) for ear infections. The ears were inflamed, discharging and smelly. She is ten years old at the time of the consultation.

Her owner explains: " Since her ears are cured she is worse. She lost all her energy; she drags behind during her walks. She seems ill, she is not interested in anything. She loves company, she is very kind, she can never have enough.

She is a good guard dog and growls when it is needed. She is not jealous but when I call one of the cats she comes up to have her share. When I push her back she is sad. She becomes lethargic in warm weather. She prefers cold weather.

She doesn't express herself, she never asks for anything, if she is thirsty she won't show this. She doesn't move; she sleeps and sleeps and sleeps.

She loves it when there are things going on in the house. When we raise our voices she is terrified. When we put her food down, she won't eat, she waits for permission. She is really passive. She never takes any initiatives.

She prefers to go for different walks, she is uninterested in ordinary walks. She likes to visit other people. The worse that can happen to her is to be excluded from the family."

The author explains how he prescribes several remedies over one year. The remedies are chosen for their 'classic' disease pictures or insufficient repertorisations (his own words).
Graphites 30K
Pulsatilla 200K
Calc carb. 30K
Sulfur 30K repeated after two weeks.
Causticum 30K
Carcinosine 200K

In between remedies, the owner loses patience and conventional treatments are given because Diane becomes stiff and finds it more and more difficult to go for her walks. Anti inflammatory medicines and later steroids don't make a big difference. She is now near a state of paralysis and a certain degree of incontinence appeared. She is duller then ever.

More comments from the owner; " She doesn't like the rain, the cold, the warmth. She likes mild temperatures and being patted. She wants everybody's affection. She has been in many households before us.

She adopted us from the first day but she felt secure in the house only after several months. She is always hungry, we have to watch her weight. This doesn't stop her from being obese and from snoring.

She is not intelligent, but she is so nice with the cats."

It is time to find a solution; Diana's quality of life is very poor. A new repertorisation is made with the following symptoms:
Suppressed eruptions, slowness, affectionate, company desire, urinating too frequently, warmth aggravates.
This produces a long list of remedies. In the 16th place Zincum is present.
One 200K dose and slowly Diane regains her normal mobility. Her ear troubles reappear for a while and recede by themselves. A few weeks later, she starts to take initiatives, which she has never done before.

It was high time to find this similimum because Diane was so bad there was talk of euthanasia. She goes on living for another two happy and dynamic years with no need for further prescriptions. She then suddenly becomes old and dies peacefully.

36) I like you, I hate you. (D Notre-Dame)

When Betty is presented for the first time she is six. She is a boxer and has suffered since the age of 6 months from a suppurating skin condition. She is covered in crusts and pustules from the nose to the tip of her tail. Where there are no crusts, there are marks of previous infections. She has been treated with antibiotics continuously since the beginning of her problems.

A lab analysis reveals the presence of a Staphylococcus Aureus resistant to most antibiotics.

Following the first consultation she receives herbal medicines and aromatherapy. This brings slight improvement but more serious medicines are needed.

After a few visits, the vet noted how, each time, Betty would come up to greet and lick him followed a few minutes later by growling and attempts to bite. Her owner confirms she is not an easy dog; she is very intolerant. On the question of where Betty sleeps, her owner answers: " She never sleeps with me, she always has refused to walk up the stairs".

This type of behaviour where liking for a person changes rapidly into dislike suggests a particular remedy. In the literature it is confirmed that this remedy is aggravated when 'ascending stairs'.

Betty receives one dose of Anacardium 30K.

This is followed by two weeks of 'evacuation of pus' via all the orifices.

One month later she receives a further dose of Anacardium MK. 95% of the pustules disappear, only some discharge in the ears remains.

One month later some symptoms reappear, another dose of the remedy, same dilution and all symptoms disappears. Betty also becomes much more happy and her aggressive character resolves itself.

Six months later, an irritating discharge from the left ear appears. This is very quickly controlled with another dose of the same remedy.

Another six months later the skin problems reappear. A conventional colleague prescribes antibiotics and steroids. This makes no difference, the skin just continues to aggravate.

Three weeks later she receives a further dose of the same homeopathic remedy, quickly followed by rapid improvement.

The odd repetition of the same remedy from time to time keeps Diane going for the following few years until she develops a paralysis and is put to sleep by a colleague on request of the owner.

37) My name is Tulip but Harmony would have suited me as well. (P Froment)

Tulip is a milking cow. She had suffered from an attack of severe mastitis three years ago. Since this episode the affection has become chronic and she needs regular antibiotic treatments to keep the infection out of her udder.

The first thing the farmer says about her is that she has a mild expression.

The inflammations go from one quarter to another. When she is not well she produces only half the usual amount of milk. She has alternating moods; they happen for no reason. "She is large and makes the others respect herself, she is not nasty. She will have mastitis and a high temperature, but continues to milk normally and eat. Last summer she had a raw inflamed patch on her udder. She allowed the farm dog to lick this wound.

One day, two cows were fighting like bulls. She came up to them and separated them quickly and efficiently. She is like an efficient policeman.

She is mild and easy going but she makes herself respected by the others without any violence.

This year her winter coat hasn't disappeared and she stays dirty. She scratches herself, she likes us to scratch her. She is the only one of the herd that lets our grand daughter approach and stroke her."

The vet notices that she has a sad look about her.

It is possible to make a repertorisation using the following symptoms: Mildness, alternating moods, itch scratching ameliorates, capriciousness.

More then 15 remedies share these symptoms. One attracts the attention of the vet: Natrum carbonicum. This remedy is associated with a desire for harmony; this explains how she establishes the order in the herd when two cows make attempts to fight.

One dose of the remedy in the 200K strength brings 'harmony' to her udder. She has no more reoccurrences of mastitis over the following two years.

38) Oops, I didn't control that. (M Brunson)

The story begins with a call out on a Sunday for abdominal cramping. Kazan is a 9 year old Doberman cross who has just moved to Europe back from Africa. He is given an allopathic treatment but because this cramping happens on a regular base, the owner is invited to make an appointment to find a long-term homeopathic remedy to help his dog.

When he comes for his first homeopathic consultation, it is the locum (also a homeopath) who sees the dog.

"It always happens the day after he has an erection; he takes the position of a sphinx, vomits his food and refuses to lie on his side. It happens every month or so. It all started 3 years ago for no apparent reason. When he has one of his crises, he likes being rubbed on the back. After the crisis he wanders around for a while.

Food does not seem to play a role. He gulps his food and when he drinks he makes a big mess. He is lean (normal for his breed) and because he is used to the African climate he likes the sun and the heat and hates the cold of our regions.

He vibes when we go out, he is afraid and worried when we take him in the car; he becomes restless and all his movements are abrupt (specially his head).

He likes playing with other dogs; he 'organises' the running with our neighbour's dog. He barks at people who are outside the garden, once inside he doesn't bother with them.

On three occasions he has bitten someone; every time in the same conditions; they brought their face close to him. This took him by surprise and he turned his head. Each time it was more of a shock than a real bite. Sometimes he holds on to people's arms without hurting them. He never announces his intentions through growling.

He loves cuddles and being stroked. He doesn't like noises; he starts to 'vibrate' and would like to hide in a mouse hole. He sometimes produces little spurts of urine.

He loves female dogs and approaches them like a car with no shock absorbers moving his hind backwards and forwards. He hates closed doors and asks us to open them. He hates cats.

When we play with him, after a while he will have an erection. This also happens when he plays with other dogs, male or female.

He is very worried when we are sad or when we lie down too long. He will come up and sniff. Sometimes he scrapes his throat followed by a swallowing effort.

He is agile and gracious. As soon as he is a few metres away from us we have no more control over him. He digs under the fence to escape."

Based on the ambience of the consultation a dose of Lycopodium 200K is administered.

Kazan is very well for four months.
When he comes to the surgery again the vet notices through the window that after Kazan emptied his bowels on the side of the drive he produced a little amount of fluid from his penis. The owner confirms later that this happens often; for instance when he receives a biscuit.

"Kazan has been well since last time but he is now always hungry. He eats anything and would burn his mouth for any food. He never drinks, he only drinks after his walks. He has bad breath.

He does not like being on his own. When he stays alone he destroys things. He is very obedient although as soon as he is a few metres away from us, we have no more control. If another dog barks at him he doesn't move, waits until the dog is passed and attacks him from behind. He likes other dogs and invites them to play."

The same remedy is repeated; you don't give up on a winning team.

Six months later Kazan is back. The second dose has made no difference at all. A friend who runs a health shop suggested a herbal treatment which he has been receiving over the last months.

A conventional colleague treated him once for 'vomiting and liver problems'. His stools have become pale, he has lost weight and started to drink copiously. He had stopped eating when Mrs and her daughter went on holiday.

After that things have been well again and he regained his weight but he is drinking more and more.
"He often trembles from excitement, from cold, when the weather changes. He still presents this fluid emission when he gets excited or when he goes to the toilet.

Every time somebody leaves the house for a period of time, he loses weight."
A blood sample at that point reveals a very high level of sugar; Kazan is diabetic. The only clinical sign is the amount he drinks and his appetite.

Normally one would expect weight loss and a few other symptoms to be present.

By using the following symptoms: urethral emission stool during, excitement during and sugar in urine, 8 remedies propose themselves. What is really unusual in this case is the absence of weakness and weight loss during diabetes. This is translated by ' absence of weakness during diarrhoea'.

Two remedies are left; Phosphoric acid and Sulfur. This case does not behave like Sulfur at all. All the affectionate behaviour, the upsets when one of the owners goes away indicate Phosphoric acid.
One dose in 30k strength and the sugar levels return to normal in a few days. No insulin treatment was necessary. Kazan finds it also much easier to cope with absences of one of his owners. He has fewer erections and the involuntary fluid emissions stopped for most of the time.

No further treatment has been necessary for two years and he now controls his 'emissions'.

39) The worm in my tail drives me mad. (P Froment)

A small queen of unknown origin is presented for nervous troubles. She attacks her tail from time to time and becomes very agitated. This alternates with phases of calmness.
A neighbour had told the elderly owners that this could be due to the presence of a worm in the tail. She received a worm tablet, which made no difference to the habit. Then the husband worried about the neighbour's tale tried to remove the worm with his knife! This only resulted in a bleeding tail; no change in behaviour.
In the consultation room the lady explained: " she is mad, you can tell by the look in her face, she is persecuted!"
Question from the vet 'what is she persecuted by?'
"It is as if there is somebody imaginary behind her. She gets angry and turns around, grabs her tail and bites it. She really goes for

herself. She wants to attack herself. When she is in the cellar she calms down. She wants to be in the cellar in the dark".

Her husband adds: "it is as if somebody imaginary is chasing her, she wants to catch somebody imaginary".

The vet decides to simply use what this old couple told him:

Delusion persecuted
Delusion pursued by enemies
Insanity, persecution mania
Mutilating his own body
Illusion injured by surroundings

Hyosciamus 200K one dose.
A fortnight later she still has the odd crisis and receives the same remedy in a higher potency. She gets worse for two days then all the symptoms disappear.

After a severe storm she gets worse again, quickly resolved by another dose of the same remedy.
She is now a normal cat and follows her owner around everywhere. They are very grateful and her tail is nicely healed.

This teaches us that it is always helpful to talk freely about one's animal without trying to be reasonable or scientific. Homeopathy can often use to great benefit any odd observations or comments on the patient which by conventional standards may seem very bizarre.

40) I am suffering but I am also cheeky. (P Froment)

Sirocco is a 6 year old pony. He is presented for laminitis. He was the grandson's riding pony but the grandson has now moved on to a bigger horse. Sirocco is still very much a favourite pet and lives a royal life in the garden of the grandparents.

As it is so often the case with ponies, Sirocco had access to too much grass; it is spring-time and he is fat. He has been stealing the grass in all the neighbours' gardens and now the vet is needed to help him with this very painful condition of the feet. He can hardly move a foot.

There is a deep friendship between this pony and his retired owners: "When I arrive and I call him he answers back with a specific noise that only we can recognise."

A conventional treatment is started and his diet is restricted.

The pain improves slowly over the next following weeks, he loses weight but he also becomes sad. He doesn't answer his owners any more.

The vet applies an old fashion treatment: a bleeding from the tips of his toes. This only makes things worse; again he doesn't want to move anymore.

The owner then accepts to seek homeopathic help.
The vet: 'Talk to me about him'

"He is a big eater, he never stops eating. He is lazy. When his belly is full he lies down and sleeps in the sun. When he goes out hacking with other horses he puts himself in front to stop the others and make them go at his pace. He is a comedian. Since his illness, when we ask him to walk he doesn't. When we have our backs turned he walks about a little"

The vet notices that he is better after he has taken a few steps.
Two remedies are given on alternate days (Ledum pallustre and Rhus tox) without much improvement after ten days.
He decides to make a proper homeopathic effort and repertorisation.

Feigns disease
Mischievous
Gluttony
Gourmand
Aggravated from rich food

Calcarea carb. is present in all these rubrics.
One dose in MK improves him for a few days but soon all goes back to the previous state.

The case needs more precision, Sirocco needs a different remedy.
'Tell me more about his comedian tricks'
" He is a comedian, he likes to tell us how unfortunate he is. He is naughty. He is very curious about noises although they startle him. He is also startled when we approach him. Last week when he refused to walk, as soon as we had our backs turned he had disappeared in the garden into eat fresh grass. When we tried to make him walk he reared."

A more appropriate repertorisation is as follows:
Liar, comedian
Mischievous
Inquisitive
Gourmand
Complaining

Veratrum album will prove a much better choice: one dose in 200K and in a week Sirocco is back to normal.
In the beginning it is his morale that improves. The owner commented: "His morale improved first, although he was still painful on his feet, he would move for us and call us. He wanted to please us. It was very strange to notice that he spontaneously walked up to us although we could see that he was still in pain".

The first thing a homeopathic (i.e. homeopathic for the patient, not just homeopathically prepared!) remedy achieves is to help the patient cope with life and his circumstances. This then gives him the freedom and possibilities to solve his health problems.

41) I am dying from nausea. (M. Brunson)

An eight week old spaniel cross is brought in the surgery for vomiting. She looks miserable. She stopped eating two days ago, and then she started vomiting.

The vomiting is accompanied by profuse salivation. She vomits large amounts. She sits up, doesn't want to lie down and has a dull expression in her eyes. She rather looks for freshness then warmth. Sometimes she drinks, sometimes she just puts her mouth in the water without drinking.

She often gags without vomiting. When she vomits, this is accompanied by lots of noises. She is in a terrible state, she has a temperature, her eyes are injected, her nose and feet are cold.

One thing strikes the vet: the amount of salivation with the vomiting.
Three doses of Ipeca 30K and 24 hours later all is well again.
Although there are several remedies that present salivating with vomiting, Ipeca is the leader of the gang in cases where vomiting brings no relief. This seemed to be the case with this puppy.
Knowing how difficult it can be to stop vomiting in dogs, this was a very successful prescription.

42) When strange observations are made often unusual remedies appear and prove effective. (P. Froment)

Sometimes the patient can be a group of animals. This time the group consists of a herd of 32 milking cows that live in a picturesque valley in southeast France. In the summer they graze the lush hillsides and in the winter they are tied up in old fashioned stables.

This herd had already benefited from homeopathic prescription 5 years prior for recurrent respiratory problems. Natrum muriaticum was a very successful remedy. The remedy had been repeated effectively several times for other problems but stopped working two years ago.

The complaint this time is lameness. It has started two years ago at the beginning of the winter. Several cows develop swelling and infection of one or more feet. This is a common affliction in cattle and caused by penetration of specific bacteria under the skin that forms the connection with the hoofs. Hygiene in this herd is managed correctly. The cattle buildings and bedding are always clean.

Vet: 'What can you say about your cows?'

Farmer: "They are stiff, they are stiff all over. It is as if the whole leg hurts. They have a good appetite. They don't want to walk on the hard soil; they choose to walk on grass or on the manure. Once they are ill they don't want to lie down. The soil seems too hard for them."

The vet observes that a few of the lame cows have a dull and dirty skin compared to the others. Their feet are red, the hoofs seem fragile and form cracks. Some of the young cows lick the soil, walls, the manure, the plastic buckets.

Vet: 'what else can you tell me?'

" The problems always arise very quickly; suddenly their legs swell up. They seem apprehensive about walking. They are reluctant to lie down, they seem to lack in space, they want to lie down further to the back where there is more soft bedding. Once they get up from lying down, their legs tremble as if they lack in strength. It seems that they have to find out how to walk."

The vet observes that during the consultation there are lots of blanks. The farmer will in a few sentences deliver a large amount of information and then suddenly stop talking for a while and even walk away to come back later.

The first three attempts are not successful (one dose of medicine is given to the entire herd)

Physostigma 30K one dose (capricious appetite and slowness walking) worked very well on two cows but not the rest of the herd.

One month later: Nux vomica (stiffness, bed seems too hard, swelling of lower limbs, dirty skin) one 200k dose. No change.

Three months later: Nitric acid 200K one dose (desire indigestible things, cracking nails, inflammation toes, resignation). No change.

Six months later, a new start of the winter: Hydrogenium 30C one dose and the winter passes without any problems. Next year, Hydrogenium 200K and all goes well again.

What made the vet decide on this remedy?
Repertorisation: sudden appearances and inflammation foot; Hydrogenium is one of the few remedies that appear. Its remedy picture contains the resignation that was sensed in the cows suffering but also the sentiment of detachment (puts things off to the following day) that was sensed in the attitude of the farmer during the consultation.
This does not mean that the farmer is the cause of the problem, it is just an example to show that if the homeopath uses anything that is peculiar or contradictory during the consultation, this may help in selecting the most appropriate remedy. In the case of a herd of milking farm animals there is often a close link between the farmer and his stock.

43) Homeopathy and prevention? (A Duport)

This farmer is a friend of the vet. She breeds ducks. For a while results are catastrophic; from 18 days of age onwards, the little ducklings start to discharge from their eyes, become dull and up to 80% die after a few days.
Of course all the usual conventional efforts have been made: autopsies, lab analysis, vaccines, hygienic measures but all this to no avail. It just gets worse over time; before shutting down the farming business a chance is given to homeopathy.

Lets observe these little ducklings: It starts with a yellow irritating discharge from the eyes. At the same time they start to limp. The lower part of their legs swells up and is filled (on autopsy) with a sticky liquid. The legs become thin. Before they die they become paralysed. Things are even worse when the weather changes.
The following symptoms produce three remedies:
Change weather aggravate
Emaciation extremities.

Dropsical swelling lower limbs
Yellow discharge from eyes
Acrid discharge from eyes

The remedies are: Arsenicum album, Carboneum sulf., Sulfur.
Sulfur is eliminated because its pathogenesis does not fit with the disease picture.

Two possible remedies: Ars.-a. and Carbn.-sulf.
It is decided to separate the candidates for treatment in two groups. One will be treated with the first remedy (group A) the other with the second remedy (group B).
At the first signs of disease in each group the remedies are administered in the drinking water.
In group A there is much less mortality but after a few days there are still a few ducklings that continue limping. In group B the symptoms disappear in one day and all the ducklings continue growing without difficulties.

Over the next year all groups of ducklings are treated with Carbon-sulf. for four days from their sixteenth day of life. Different dilutions (4C, 9C, 15C and 30C) produce similar results.
After one year of successful 'prevention' it is decided to continue with the 30C dilution and progressively stop all the conventional prophylaxis like preventive worming and 3 types of vaccines (Typhose, Cholera and Derzy). The remedy is given to the ducklings between the age of 15 and 18 days.
All goes well and after conventional prophylaxis was stopped food conversion (relation of the amount of food consumed and the gain in weight) and quality of ducks improved.

Three years down the line the homeopathic treatments are stopped. Very soon the symptoms reappeared again. As soon as the remedy was re-administered all returned back to normal.

Five years later the remedy is stopped again with no relapse of the symptoms this time.

Four years later the feedback from the farm says that all is still going well.

This case shows clearly that prophylaxis with homeopathy is possible but only if you know what the symptoms of the disease are. The advantage of treating these types of animal groups is that the external factors don't change much from year to year. New generations are issued from the mothers that originate from the flock; even genetically there is not much change. As a consequence the way disease expresses itself in such groups can be fairly constant. This explains why the same remedy was so successful over this long period.

Always be reminded that it is the symptoms that indicate an appropriate remedy not some rationale that justifies the use of a homeopathic prepared substance based on a scientific finding.

44) A countryside tale. (P Polis)

The weather was murky and November already well advanced. The rain hadn't stopped since the previous day. When, in the evening, the farmer braved the weather to inspect 9 of his young stock grazing in the hills, 8 of them ran off as usual, the ninth did not get up and stayed where she was without moving as much as an eyelid.

He walked up close to her and with a convincing use of the tip of his boot managed to make her rise. She staggered. With a great deal of difficulties he managed to make her walk to the protection of the nearby stables.

When the vet arrives, she is laid down in a corner in fresh straw. She does not pay any attention to the entry of this dreaded stranger. Even when the vet starts to examine her she does not move a hair. She feels cold and is in hypothermia.

In the light of a torch, a minute continuous movement of the head is observed, her eyes are fixed and the pupils dilated. When a finger is moved dangerously close to her eyes, she only blinks when the finger touches the cornea - she is blind.

'Hmm hmm' says the vet.
"She has caught a cold", adds the farmer.

Several new efforts by vet and farmer to make her rise prove unsuccessful; only the loud barking of the farmer's mongrel finally convinces her to get up.

Then the vet proceeds to what most farm vets do; examine rectally. When after a short examination he retracts his arm, a small amount of gelatinous, yellow-clear, sticky mass escapes from her bum.

Our patient then takes a few steps, kneels down on her front legs and stays for a while in this position with her head on the floor until she decides on what side she would lie.

The vet makes the following repertorisation:
Mind indifferent to everything
Head motions involuntary
Stool mucus, jelly, tenacious, transparent

She receives a dose of Helleborus 30C and a warm glucose drip.

Later at night when the worried farmer visited his sick animal he was happy to see her jumping up and produce a healthy amount of urine as soon as he entered the stable.

The next day she was chewing her cud again; all was well until five days later. She was lying down again, head low, indifferent to everything, still blind.

The farmer rings the vet again. Is this a sad moment after a brilliant success?

A few granules of the same remedy in 200K are cautiously hidden in the patient's mouth.

The next morning she is up and eating again.

It will take about a month for her eyesight to come back to normal but when she comes in from pasture 12 months later she is as pretty and fat as all her fellow cows and has no problems finding her way around.

And the farmer comments: "She doesn't like the cold, as soon as it rains she arches her back"

Homeopathy can cure the consequences of a cold but that doesn't mean the patient is never going to feel the cold any more.

45) Tafeta's worries and her family. (M Brunson)

It is usually nice to see a litter of young puppies arriving in the consultation room. It is worrying and sad when they are 12 days old and it is reported that over a few days one after another they have died. One died the first day, one the second, one the fourth and one the eleventh day. Four of the boxer puppies are left. The prospect of them surviving is not brilliant; puppy fading syndrome has a poor prognosis.

The first three puppies were found dead without any signs of disease. They seem to die in inverse order to that in which they were born. The sixth puppy is the weakest in the remaining litter; she is lethargic and isolates herself. Urgent action is needed.

Vet: 'What can you tell me'?

This question is followed by a long silence. There is nothing to say about the puppies, they are just puppies, like normal puppies. In such cases it is possible to use the symptoms of the mother.

Vet: 'Tell me about Tafeta'.

"She has changed since her mating. This was her first mating. She refrained from eating for two days after her mating; she was strange and seemed worried. She did the same just before she started whelping.

When the puppies were born she was clumsy with them. She still does not really want to stay with them, she leaves them alone and goes away. She growls if one of the other dogs approaches them. She seems happier and lively when she is with the other dogs.

Normally she is very peaceful. She always seems warm; she will always lie on the cold tiles.

The whelping has took a long time; she was rather thin. She had found it difficult to eat at the end because her abdomen was so full. When her puppies cry she doesn't respond."

Restless, anxious, neglects her own children, jealousy, warm aggravate
Lycopodium is chosen over Pulsatilla, Kali carb., Nux v. and Camphora
    A dose of the 12C potency is given to the puppies: four times the first day, three times the second and two times the third day
A 200K dose is given twice the first day to the mother.

The two sick puppies recuperate rapidly and none of the others become sick.
The bitch calms down and rapidly starts to behave like a normal mother.
The mother and the remaining pups enjoy a normal time and successful weaning.

This is another example of successful treatment for very young animals based on the symptoms of the mother. This system works very well as long as the strong natural bond between mum and offspring is still present; when the babies are still very dependent on their mother.

46) A phone-call for a cure. (M Brunson)

This farmer calls only sporadically; only when he is in real trouble does he call on the homeopathic vet to sort out the problems.

One of his six months old, very valuable calves developed pneumonia a week ago. Antibiotics have not made any difference.

The consultation is done over the phone because the farm is situated 100 miles away from the vet's practice.

The farmer explains: "She salivates when she is tied up. She goes to the drinking basin but it is unclear how much she drinks. She eats in the morning but not in the evening. She holds her head low and keeps away from the others. She is always wet on her back. She has a short cough every time she moves; she is afraid to cough.

Normally she is very nervous, rather frightened. Her stools are dry."

Afraid to cough, progressive pneumonia, dry stools, Bryonia imposes as a remedy. A 30K dose three times per day and three days later all is well again.

Sometimes homeopathy gives the impression of being really simple.

47) Mild medicine for serious problems. (M Brunson)

The same farmer this time is in a real panic! A group of 12 calves have shown symptoms of pneumonia since noon. They developed high fevers.

"They all seem drugged and walk around slowly or lean against the barriers of the pen. Others are standing in front of the support beams of the stable without moving as if hypnotised. The worst affected are salivating. They started coughing yesterday. Their backs are wet. Most of them make only small, rapid respiration motions. The weather has just changed to mild and rainy - well it is raining cats and dogs."

This group of animals represents an important capital amount for the farmer. When a week ago he had a similar problem with another group, they were less affected by the pneumonia. When he injected them with antibiotics they got worse. A few of them collapsed and three died. He is reluctant to inject this lot with antibiotics; he wants a kind and efficient medicine.

Intense heat, sudden appearance, dullness heat during, perspiration during fever, salivation during heat.

Belladonna 30K is administered every 3 hours.

In 48 hours 11 of the twelve are back to normal. The 12th calf received a few other remedies but then needed the help of an antibiotic injection to get over his pneumonia.

48) I like it hot but I don't mind the cold. (J P Spillbauer)

When Hooch comes in for a homeopathic consultation, he receives a daily steroid dose for his allergic skin condition. Blood analysis showed sensitivity to fleas, house dust and mites.
When the allergic condition expresses itself, Hooch loses appetite, his eyes become red, the right ear and his private parts become inflamed.

Before going down the road of more steroids and desensibilisation (immunotherapy), the owner prefers to try homeopathy.

Listen to what the owner has to say about her dog: "I bought him at 2 and a half months from a reputable breeder; he has excellent origins. His problems started four months ago; red patches developed on his abdomen.

He is a nice dog but he dominates our other dog Puli who is the older one. He drinks, eats and gets in the car before her. He is afraid of nothing. He likes other dogs but he tries to dominate them. He likes children and usually gives them licks. Our garden is like a battlefield; he tosses everything about. He sleeps in the corridor with his head under the radiator, which is switched on and very hot. He will stay outside the whole day without any problems.

He behaves very bossily with Puli; it seems that he gives her orders; he forces her to sleep on the sofa.
It has taken him a long time before he got used to his name but he was clean very young."

During the consultation Hooch slept along a wall of the room and seemed indifferent to what was going on in the room. When the consultation is finished he walks out as if nothing has happened.

Warm stove ameliorates, dictatorial and forgets his own name suggest Camphora as a remedy. One 30C dose is given.

A month later the skin is much better and so are ears and eyes. His owner is very pleased and calls the improvement 'spectacular'.

"Hooch still keeps to himself, he is still dominant. He has refused to enter the train station where I wanted to weigh him"

No remedy: wait. Steroids were stopped one week after the dose.

Five months later.

"He has been very well. A few days ago the allergy came back. The skin is red, wet and discharging. He has an awful smell. Generally he is well in himself.

He is more obedient now and calmer in the car. Before it was impossible to transport him. He is very playful but still dominant. Three weeks after previous treatment he became much easier to train.

Three days ago we applied an anti-parasitic substance on the carpets and floors."

Hooch receives a new dose of Camphora, this time in a XM K dilution.

His skin problems regress in a few days and he becomes more respectful.

Six months later he develops hemorrhagic stools (non-diarrheic) and refuses to eat after having ingested a buffalo skin toy. He looks for cool places to lie down. He passed a very agitated night.

It is remarkable to discover these symptoms during an acute problem caused by the ingestion of a 'foreign body': they are typical symptom associated with the remedy Camphora. A 200K dose puts everything quickly back in place.

The owner confirms again how much easier it has become to control his dog.

49) His curiosity wins over his condition. (JP Spillbauer)

It is always when cases are desperate that they arrive in the homeopathic surgery. Luckily for the patients, homeopathy is a powerful tool when a serious effort is made.

When Poppers is presented to the vet he is just six years old but only one step away from euthanasia. He has been kept alive by a colleague with drips and lots of injections; when a cat's urea level has been above 3 grams for four weeks the prognosis is very poor. A kidney transplant seems to be the only possibility to save him.

Poppers has been a regular client at the vets. He developed an allergy that started under his chin and later developed all over his head. He lost the fur on his face. A specialist in dermatology advised to treat him more or less continuously with steroids.

At some point he also developed a circulatory problem on one of his posteriors. Anti-coagulants managed the symptoms but he lost two toes in the battle.

Before his kidney problems started, his owner had just started a new steroid treatment for reoccurring skin allergy.

Although he has a very high urea level he still eats a little. He spends the day prostrated in a corner when once he was continually playing. Before the kidney troubles started he was licking the walls, a flowerpot, cement and soil. This caused frequent vomiting.

The owner explains: "He is a very kind, playful and affectionate cat. He changed overnight after we had him castrated. He became more sociable. Before his castration he didn't play and went to hide when somebody came in the house. After his castration he could not get enough from playing, he was forever trying to make us run behind him. He also played endlessly with his toys.

When he urinated he always got up before he finished and therefore finished his puddle outside the cat litter tray. He is obstinate and capricious. He would ask for something to eat and then refused it to finish his dish during the night."

The vet notices how much weight he lost but regardless of his severe state he jumped off the table to explore the consultation room. Although he seemed anxious he continued examining all the corners of the room. "His curiosity always wins over his fears", adds his owner. As soon as he is lifted on the table, he jumps off again and continues his explorations. When a dog enters the surgery, Popper walks up to the glass door and has a good look at what is happening.

The symptoms,
> Desire for lime etc.
> Inquisitive
> Playful

don't really produce an interesting remedy.

What strikes the vet is the indifference of Poppers to his condition: he should be dull and lying around instead of exploring the consulting room considering the bad state of his kidneys.

He then chooses two other rubrics:
> Anxiety walking ameliorates
> Indifferent to suffering, to his condition

Only one remedy comes out: Scorpion. This remedy is not available and is considered an error in the literature. Two other scorpions are available: Buthus australicus and Androctonus.

But-a. is given twice per day in the 7C strength.

In a few days time, the urea level drops and Poppers 'becomes more relaxed' explains his owner. The remedy is stopped after two weeks when Poppers started playing again.

His blood urea goes down to more acceptable levels.

Poppers lives well for five months. Then his owner telephones to say that a colleague has put him to sleep and thanked us for the extra happy months they enjoyed.

Poppers did not benefit from a further homeopathic prescription before or when things got bad again. We will never know whether it would have been possible to make him continue enjoying his life. This is a common occurrence because conventional knowledge finds it difficult to accept what homeopathy can realise and cases are quickly considered incurable or too desperate to pursue.

50) Talking about unusual remedies. (E De Beukelaer)

Tigrou, a spayed queen of unknown origin, came to see me for the first time at the age of two in April 2000.

She had a blackish slightly sticking discharge from both ears, the side of mouth and between her toes. The main complaint was a persistent licking under her abdomen, under her four legs and under her tail causing the skin to become red and weeping from infection.

(This type of skin complaint in cats is called nervous grooming and is the expression of some underlying behavioural problem/anxiety)

There are a few skin crusts on her back.

She had chronic ear complaints when she first came to the house at the age of four months. Many different allopathic and homeopathic treatments made no difference until at the age of nine months the symptoms receded following the use of juniper healing oil. She was spayed at the age of 8 months.

Let's listen to what the owner told me:

"She is a very mild cat, she is slightly clumsy and doesn't show the normal 'tricky' cat behaviour. I call her my dog-cat. She is not influenced by the seasons. She never surprises me. She is a little awkward and makes things fall over. She likes company and sleeps against me at night but never wants to stay on my lap for more than a few seconds. She has difficulties in accepting strangers; she avoids them as much as possible. Sometimes she looks as if she has seen a monster. She doesn't like to be manipulated. She is very timid. She is very easily scared; she seems permanently scared since we moved into our new house. I have never seen her drink. She has always been in the background but she is now really paranoid. She always has her ears folded backwards, 'where can I hide?' If I come up behind her she is frightened."

After this first and then a second consultation I make the following prescriptions:
Ambra grisea, a month later Baryta carbonicum followed a month later by Pulsatilla. The remedies don't make any difference, neither does a long course of antibiotics and the use of Feliway (appeasing pheromone).

Fourth consultation in September 2000. Things were getting worse!

The owner speaks again: "She is in a hurry to go from one place to an other, she always has an expression of fear, sometimes she just lays in a corner or in the middle of the corridor like a bag of dirty linen".
The owner reminds me of the blackish discharge from her mouth corners, ears and paws. The discharge is really abundant, that is not a common symptom.

I check in the repertory and find the following symptom:

Perspiration, bloody,

My eye spotted a remedy I had just learned about; its fear from society, 'he wants to escape from society because he knows he does something wrong (Jeremy Sherr)'. The remedy is Canabis indica.
There was my cat-'junky' lying like a heap of dirty linen, kicking off her last 'trip'. The remedy gave me an explanation for the unusual comment my client made about how she looked like a bag of dirty linen.

Cannabis indica 9C twice in 12 hours was administered.

The first ten days nothing really happened and then gradually the behaviour improved and she stopped licking. Three months later the skin is completely healed and the fur is growing back. Tigrou is still very shy but adapted finally to a new kitten that arrived in the summer. She now has a more normal cat behaviour.
When I saw her again in July 2001, everything was still going fine. No further medicine was needed.

51) A quick prescription with unexpected results. (E De Beukelaer)

Tequila came to see me for the first time when she was 11 months old. She is a Belgian Shepherd cross bitch and had been treated by a colleague with steroids and non steroidal medicines since the age of four months for lameness of the hind legs. It started off with the one but then the other hip became painful as well.

An X-ray showed important changes in the hip joints; the future of this poor little pup did look rather bleak. When the colleague suggested that an ablation of the femur heads (first the one then the other) would be the only way to reduce the pain, the owner had come to us to try something else first.

I asked the owner to tell Tequila's story: "When she arrived at four months she was already limping. Everything got worse when our vet manipulated her hips when he examined her.

She doesn't want to eat anymore since the painkillers have lost their initial efficiency. She stays in her bed and loses weight.
Before she was much more of an outdoor dog. She is afraid when we shout. She doesn't like it when the children quarrel. She is very sweet. She is very patient with the children and only barks what is necessary. She doesn't like the car.

The severe pains, she is feeling now, started one evening."

When I examine her she doesn't complain. She doesn't complain when she is handled in the house either.

" She doesn't like the cold and sleeps close to the radiator or in the sun. She will keep the painful leg up from the morning to the evening. Since she is in pain she sleeps on our bed. She doesn't like cheese"

What was striking in this observation is the lassitude with the pain. The owner had talked about the vivacity of Tequila during her first few months. By hearing how she has been over the last weeks and by looking at her in the consultation room, it strikes me how 'down' she is with the pain. Most young dogs put up with hip pain, especially when there is no real reaction to the manipulation of the hip during the consult. The pain doesn't appear to be that important.

Looking through the repertory I stumble on a symptom that reads: 'Discouraged from pain'. Nux vomica is one of the remedies present. I am at the beginning of my homeopathic career and think by myself that Nux vomica is used by many homeopaths as a 'cleansing substance' for the consequences of overuse of allopathic medicine. Tequila's list of medicines was longer than my arm, so I thought that a little course of Nux vomica would do her some good.

She takes Nux vomica 5C once per day for 5 days.

When I see her again a week later for further prescription, I cannot recognise the puppy I met earlier. She had gained weight and was much more bouncier. She received one more dose of Nux vomica 7C during the consultation.

Until I lost contact when Tequila was three years old, she never took any other medicine for lameness of the hind legs and had the most enjoyable life.

Such cases show how generous homeopathic medicine can be. As long as there is an observation that has homeopathic value (the lassitude, unusual for this breed, that was clearly observed and expressed by the owner) the chance of finding an extremely efficient remedy is great even when the justification for the prescription is not very homeopathic (using a remedy for draining purposes). This case also shows that not only high dilutions are efficient; WHAT COUNTS IS GIVING THE RIGHT REMEDY!

I remember a case presented in a congress in Belgium: the patient was an immigrant who worked hard for many years suffering with severe backaches without complaining until his children were all settled in their adult life. Only then he allowed himself to afford a consultation with a homeopathic doctor (after having spend many useless consultations in conventional hospitals). The homeopath was astonished by the calm acceptance of his suffering; he received one dose of Ignatia 7C. (Accepts the most severe suffering without complaining) The case was presented two years after the dose which had not been repeated since. All his back pains had disappeared in a few weeks.

52) Life is horrible to me. (E. De Beukelaer)

Tess really exaggerates, she is a mare that is not easy to handle. Her father was known for producing fillies with a difficult character but Tess, even at 12, is still quite a handful. I must say that she hadn't had an easy life. Her owner rescued her from a place where she was stabled in very poor conditions with the sole purpose of fattening and being sold for butchery. Not a nice beginning to life! She had witnessed many of her friends disappearing forever.

Then follows a long list of illnesses, all treated with allopathic medicines. She started with respiratory diseases followed by regular attacks of colic, repeating themselves more and more often (she has been turned inside out in the Veterinary College of Ghent, but they found nothing abnormal). Every time, one administration of antispasmodic treatment was sufficient to calm the storm. Then the excesses of colic are replaced with tying up syndromes (inflammation of the large muscle masses). When these happen she is completely blocked and cannot move at all. They mostly happen during the small walks she has in the neighbourhood when she suddenly takes fright for no apparent reasons.

Tess is really lucky to have the most patient and determined owner in the world who is not afraid of horses because Tess regularly tries to take command.

When we decide to search for a homeopathic solution for her ongoing problems, the main complaints are the recurring panic attacks for no apparent reason. She will either rear up and become really restless or tie up and become extremely difficult to move for several hours (or days). When she becomes 'blocked' outside the property where she lives, she will only move to go back to her stable. This happens mostly when they (Tess and her owner) go out for one of their daily walks around the block of pastures and houses but can also happen when she is grazing in a corner of her paddock. During or after these attacks she will sometimes start to graze frenetically. Very often her hind legs tremble and she sweats copiously.

She is aggressive with everybody except her owner because she demands to be respected.

She has a maternal instinct. She used to defend a foal with which she was in the field for a while.

Tess received the typical 'fear' remedies.
Opium worked quite well for six months, then nothing anymore. Aconite, Sulf-acid and Argentum nitricum didn't make any difference. This is not surprising because I didn't ask: what is peculiar in this case, what is special in this case. I just tried the remedies that have a renowned efficiency for cases where fear is an important ingredient.

What is typical in this case is how Tess over-reacts all the time; she really exaggerates all her reactions: all the physical symptoms always look very severe although they never cause any real chronic or severe medical conditions; the 'severe' colic signs are always very quickly treated with a simple anti-spasmodic injection. She had a rough time when she was younger.

The remedy that covers this is Chamomille. One 200K dose transformed her. All her annoying complaints disappeared. She is still a little difficult to handle but nothing compared to before. She received a further 1M dose 8 months later for re-occurrence of some of the symptoms and 5 years down the line she is still doing well.

53) Either I sleep or I convulse. (A Duport)

This little 7 week old West Highland White terrier is presented in emergency one Saturday evening; she is convulsing very badly.

The first crisis happened a week before. She had vomited a large quantity of worms. She was consequently wormed and received a few antispasmodic pills over four days.

When she is brought into the surgery, she was having her third crisis in a few hours time. As soon as we approach her she takes a sternal position, her jaw starts to clack rapidly, she howls, her eyelids tremble. Within ten seconds she then turns on her back and continues to convulse and cry while she pedals with her legs. She passes a small amount of stools and urinates abundantly during the crisis.

After the crisis she gets up and turns around in a circle for five minutes. She then gets tired and falls asleep. He pupils are widely open but she does not respond to her surroundings.

As soon as she is touched, the same scenario reproduces itself until she falls asleep again.

She is given a few granules of Causticum 30C because she turned around to the right each time (vertigo, turning to the right).

She is left quiet over night but in the morning it is obvious that the treatment had not made any difference.

After a good night's sleep the vet reckoned that his head was much clearer; that was a good thing because a different remedy is needed.

The following symptoms are used: Sleep between epileptic crises, convulsions falling on back and urination during convulsions. One of the remedies present is Oenanthe.

After a quick check in the Materia Medica of Allen it is obvious that this may be a more suitable remedy.

She receives one 15C tablet. When she has a new fit one hour later she didn't cry during the crisis. She has a mild crisis in the afternoon and seems to respond to visual stimuli again. She has a meal in the evening and goes home the following day.

She will have one more crisis the fifth day and thereafter settles to a normal life. Over the following years she never presented any more fits.

54) A homeopathic tranquilliser? No, an appropriate remedy. (P Rouchossé)

Two days ago, Balcane a big dairy cow slipped, fell on her head and broke off her left horn.

When the vet attends the animal, she is disfigured: she is left with a very sore bloody stump where the right horn was broken off. She has a high temperature, is very lethargic and pus is coming out of the nostril on the side of the broken horn. The infection has penetrated into one of the sinuses, no wonder she is not feeling well.

The vet decides to remove the damaged piece of horn to be able to clean out the wound and the infected sinus.

Balcane decides differently! Even after having received a huge dose of tranquilliser, there is no way she lets anyone approach her very painful head. She becomes very agitated as soon as the horn or her head is touched. The vet even suspects a touch of meningitis due to the severity of the agitation.

Luckily the farmer is a convinced customer of homeopathy and asks the vet to use homeopathy rather then conventional techniques.

Three symptoms:

Constitutional effects of wounds
Injuries of the head
Septic fever

One dose of Arnica 30C, and 24 hours later all is well.

Homeopathy does not need to be complicated, but even arnica works better when it is properly selected for the case based on the patient's symptoms.

55) The wart that convinced the disbeliever. (J Dabeux)

One of his colleague friends who is rather sceptical about the vet's homeopathic activities reluctantly refers his own dog. The 4 year old, cross breed bitch has a wart on her left elbow. He has to admit his failing; he already has surgically removed a wart on this location twice and used many local and general treatments to no avail.

Every time the wart grew back very quickly and is now getting bigger every month. She scratches it until it bleeds.

A little hesitatingly he agrees to say a few words about Laïka: "She is calm but she is the leader over our other male dog. For two and a half years she has been receiving injections to stop her coming on heat.

She doesn't like the cold. When she goes out in the cold she loses all her energy. She eats well, but she doesn't like changes being made in her diet. She swells up easily when stung by insects. She is very obedient and friendly with us."

It is difficult to obtain good homeopathic symptoms from a sceptical, conventional vet, but he has been kind enough to say a few interesting words.

The following symptoms are used:

Warm stove ameliorates, menses suppresses, intolerant of contradiction (change of food) warts on upper limbs and must scratch until it bleeds.

Arsenicum album comes out strongest and is given twice in a 30C dilution two weeks apart.

Three weeks later the wart was gone and all the fur was growing back. A few months later his friend told him that Laïka was less susceptible to the cold. Laïka lost her wart and he lost some of his scepticism on the subject of homeopathy.

56) I will help you if you protect me. (B Heude)

Initially, Junior was named Helios by the breeder. This was a rather pretentious name; Junior was not the proud German Shepherd he should be. His ears were too long and floppy, his tail was too long and his body disproportionate. Sadly he was a true representation of the quality of the breeder's standards.

His owner is an energetic nurse who lives with her 90 year old mother.

The allergic skin condition in his both ears make his life very unpleasant. Nevertheless, his owner takes him regularly to the local dog club for training.

The consultation starts with the following question: Talk to me about his character?

"Until he was one year old he was very anxious, he was afraid in the dark, I needed to accompany him. I forced him to go in the dark on his own and the fear has disappeared."

This owner doesn't talk easily; the vet has to re-launch the consultation several times by asking a question.

What is he afraid of?

"He doesn't like people who talk loudly or are exuberant. He doesn't like others to stroke him; he trembles and goes away. Even at the club where he knows everybody, he comes close to me and trembles with fear when people insist on stroking him. He is never into trouble. When his litter mates were fight playing he got out of the way, he has always preferred the quiet.

He is calm in everything he does. He eats calmly. From the beginning we have put his bowl in the middle of a little rug to prevent him making a mess on the floor. When it is dinnertime he fetches the rug. Once we forgot to take the rug on holiday; he refused to eat.

He doesn't like sweets, cakes and other dainties and refuses to drink milk. We have to melt some butter on his vegetables otherwise he won't eat them. He likes salami but refuses to eat fish in any form.

He takes his time in everything he does. He is phlegmatic and never gets worked up, even when he plays. He is afraid of people. Traffic and fireworks don't worry him. He is worried when I go out, he doesn't mind when my mother goes away.

The warmth in the summer affects him. He likes a cover in the winter but he does not sleep in front of the radiators. He hates water, he hates going out when it rains and walks around puddles."

What was the most difficult point in his training?

"He takes a while to learn things, but once acquired it stays."

How is he with bitches?

"He is not interested at all, even when they are in heat"

What is the most annoying part of his character?

"He is slow in everything, it takes time for him to assimilate things. He is easy and always in the same good mood. He never shows any joy"

How is he with your mother?

"When she is tired and falls asleep on the sofa, he will lie by her side on the floor"

How is he with you, would he defend you?

"He would be worried for my mother and protect her, with me it is different. If there is a noise at night he comes up to my room to wake me and then makes me understand that I have to solve the problem myself and walks off again"

What is peculiar in this case? The modalities are not very precise apart from food preferences. What is clear is his attitude to danger: help me when I am in trouble, take care of yourself when I don't sense any danger.

Other clear feature is his slowness to learn (slow to learn to talk)

He receives one dose of Causticum 200K. The eczema disappears and he becomes more self-assured.

(There is two years of feed back with no further need for medicines after this prescription)

57) I suffer quietly. (E De Beukelaer)

This little orange coloured canary was the latest expensive acquisition of a client who has just returned to breeding after having been ten years without his beloved birds. She was still in quarantine when she was mated. She wasn't supposed to accept the male bird she was caged with because it was not the mating season (September)!

Anyway: she is nesting, but no eggs appear. Her abdomen is swollen but no egg is visible in the cloaca. This is a serious condition in these small birds.

The application of liquid paraffin did not make any difference. The only consequence is that the poor little bird spent the whole day yesterday cleaning the oily stuff off its feathers.

Surgical removal of the egg is possible but not without substantial risk.

In the morning and evening she goes to her nest to try and pass her egg but every time she gives up after a few attempts. She is still happy and eats well. When her cage is put on the consultation table, she is not worried like most of my other patients; she sits there still washing off some of the liquid paraffin on her feathers.

The following symptoms are used:
Ailments from homesickness (comes on heat the wrong time of year, after arriving in her new home), slow delivery, labour pains ceasing

Ignatia 200K is dissolved in water. She receives a drop during the consultation and a drop later in the evening. The following day she lays a very large egg, which hatches successfully.

58) Irritable is an appropriate adjective for Gigi. (JP Spillbauer)

'Help me or I will bite you' seems to scream out Gigi a 5 year old sterilised queen. She was adopted when she was two.

"She sits on our lap, quietly. As soon as we start to stroke her, her tail starts to sway, she bites us but she will stay on our lap. She is calm and nervous at the same time"

Gigi has always been like this.

"She always attacks one of our other cats. When I try to protect this cat, she will attack me and bite me severely; she will dangle off my hand her teeth deeply imbedded in it."

It is only Mrs who receives this treatment. Her husband has never been bitten. He has always been allowed to play with her.

The reason for the consultation is an elevated blood uraemia reading and mild increased liver values over the past few months. Allopathic treatment for liver and kidney problems produce no results.

"She is often agitated and nervous. She goes in and out the house. As soon as something isn't right she agitates her tail; several times she has made things fall off the table with her tail. In the car she sits happily on Mrs' lap. As soon after she has bitten me or terrorised the other cat she becomes calm again.

She has no physical problems. She doesn't run around everywhere, she doesn't climb trees, she plays normally. When we touch her she becomes tense and feels hard. She has no fear.

She is very peaceful with all the other cats apart from the one she will aggravate from time to time. She will stalk him and then attack him. He is a 16 year old cat with only one eye who is not dominant at all. She really bites him to hurt him out of anger.

When friends come, she will sit on everybody's lap, whipping her tail. She will put her teeth on their hands to say stop but she never bites them.

Strange cats do not bother her; she even allows them to eat from her bowl! At the vet's she is OK to be treated but when we try to give her a tablet she shreds us to pieces."

The vet notices the strange difference between the kind behaviour of this cat in the consult room and the horror stories that are told on her behalf; when Mrs picks her up from the basket in the consultation room she purrs happily.

First prescription: Anacardium. The remedy makes no difference.

Several other prescriptions will follow to no effect. (Nitric acid, Lycopodium, Belladonna, Stramonium)

The following consultations always bring back a similar story: "She wants to be with me but as soon as I show some affection, she bites me and attacks the other cat. If I defend the other cat she will turn around me and bite my ankles or my hands. As soon as she has bitten me her agitation stops. The other cat is terrorised. I wonder if it is her liver problem that affects her behaviour. She is all right with other people and will only mildly grab them with her teeth. She will jump on to my shoulder and be really friendly. Then suddenly she will bite me.

What is strange is that she seems calm and at the same time her tail will be whipping in a sign of agitation."

Hepar sulfur, repeated several times, brings some improvement. "Gigi is still agitated but with a lower intensity when she attacks, she bites with much less intensity". Not much of an improvement.

Signs of seborrhoea on the base of her tail appeared. The blood values for liver and kidneys don't change. She has very bad breath: the remedy is not right.

Her owner repeats: "Maybe her character is affected by her liver problem?
She is friendly with all the other cats, one of them is in love with her, she accepts all his attentions. She never bites anyone else"

Many remedies have been used following many different symptom selections for repertorisations, until the vet realised that in three different consultations, the owner made the same remark: "Could her character change have to do with her liver problems?"
In the repertory there is a rubric that sounds as follows: 'Irritability in liver trouble'. Four remedies are present: Bryonia, Chamomilla, Nux-vomica and Podophyllum.
After reading the Materia Medica of each of these remedies, one dose of Chamomilla 30C is administered.
Three weeks later her owner reported that she had improved at all levels. Even the behaviour towards the other cat improved. But a few days ago, she started vomiting and her breath became smelly again. Her aggressiveness reappeared and she had diarrhoea.
A dose of Chamomilla XMK is administered.
This time the improvement is lasting. Her behaviour towards Mrs and the other cat has become completely normal. Her blood values returned to normal and she started to play again as when she was younger. Several years later she is still fine.

We do recognise Chamomilla in this case, like in the case of Tess and the calf with diarrhoea; exaggerated behaviour.

59) I am chicken, I hide. (A Duport)

These poor young chicks should be happy to live in an organic farm. Their advantageous living conditions don't seem to stop them developing the same annoying diseases as their mates in conventional farms. This group of 4 weeks old produces the classical signs of coccidiosis; semi liquid stools with a little blood and arrest in weight gain. What is different from their colleagues in conventional farms is that they are not allowed the usual drugs to stop these parasites from developing in their intestines.

The homeopathic vet is called out to the farm. He asks the classic 'homeopathic' question: "What have you noticed special in this lot compared to what you usual see with your poultry?"

"The diarrhoea is brownish, they don't grow, sometimes there is some blood in the diarrhoea".

Vet: 'Well yeah, that is all the normal stuff, anything peculiar?'

Farmer: "What is strange is that they seem to hide. Some find it difficult to stay on their legs, their legs are weak" The vet then observes for himself that, indeed, they seem to bend down and hide their heads under straw and dead leaves that lie on the ground. "They don't want to be looked at but it seems that they observe us from the corner of their eyes" adds the farmer.

That is really strange, it seems as if all the chicks in the group behave like this.

In the repertory there is a rubric that says: Gestures, covering face with hands, but looking through their fingers, in children.

One of the remedies present is Baryta carb.

Hiding from fear, dwarfishness and weakness of legs are also symptoms that belong to this remedy.

They receive the remedy in 30C in the drinking water for three days.

From day two they are much better. They make up their setback and finish their cycle in good health without the need for any vitamins or other medicines.

Concerning the hiding game, this stopped from the next day because all the dead leaves were removed by the farmer.

Conclusion: even poultry can express behaviour symptoms that are useful for successful homeopathic prescription. Never be afraid to make any comment to your homeopath. Nothing is without importance.

60) Clandestine distillation. (A Duport)

The comments of this farmer on his two days old calf are very concise: "It seems that his bladder is full but have you noticed the prune juice he distils, it even looks like it liberates hot fumes, burning his...(countryside expression for anus)"

The calf lies on his side, doesn't want to drink, is in hypothermia and has an enlarged, gas filled abdomen. The diarrhoea smells awful and several of his joints are swollen. Things could not be worse.

Two symptoms: swelling of joints and stool watery like prune juice.

They produce two remedies: Arsenicum album and Terebintina.

Terebentina 30C, given three times in two hours liberates an abundant amount of gas and hemorrhagic stools of the most smelly kind. Then the calf gets up and goes to his mum to have his first drink in 36 hours. Problem solved without any other medicines.

Remember: diarrhoea does not always means Arsenicum album as it is often recommended.

61) Locked in spasms. (J Dabeux)

Intensive selection techniques have created a type of cattle called Belgian Blue. This breed is known for its hypertrophied musculature. More muscles means more meat! This is a much appreciated quality for the farming world but intensive selecting often also brings side effects with it. At first, most of the cows find it difficult to give birth normally and have to undergo a Caesarean section for every calf. Once they are born they can still be affected with several problems typical of the breed.

One of these afflictions is a contraction of the Achilles muscle mass. This muscle mass will contract as soon as the calf puts his feet on the floor and causes his hind leg to throw itself spasmodically backwards. This happens regularly in young calves but can be successfully operated on.

That is exactly what happened to this 7 months old Belgian Blue calf. He has been fine since he was operated on five months ago.

Over the last week, he finds it difficult to get up and mostly lies on the ground. As soon as he rises, his legs become contracted and rigid. He will only stand up for five seconds and then lie down again. When he lies down he is fine and eats and drinks normally.

He has grown more or less normally since his operation.

"Since he was young, he always has been a fearful calf. As soon as we or somebody else comes in the stable, he jumps up out of fear and trembles all over. When he is approached he has a wild and fearful look on him."

Symptoms selected: Starting from fright, facial expression wild, shortened muscles and tendons, standing impossible, trembling upper and lower limbs.

They produce the following remedies: Nitric acid, Hyosc., Plumbum, Mercurius, Opium, Stramonium, Conium and Cuprum.

Plumbum metallicum is preferred.

30C four times for two days. He improves.

MK (one dose) the third day and after a few days, he can stand up. He is still weak and falls over regularly.

XMK one week later (one dose) he improves further and returns to normal. His previous anxiety also improved significantly.

62) Like in a fairy tale; the toad becomes princess (again). (M. Brunson)

I was elected vice-champion of Europe in Brussels a few months ago in a best milking cow contest. I am proud, pretty, elegant and tall. My keeper is very proud of me, he talks about me all the time and even refused the £ 15,000 a German farmer offered for me.

But a few days after the contest, a nasty form of mastitis developed in my body parts so much admired. It started in one quarter but soon spread to all quarters. After lengthy treatments with antibiotics and steroids, the milk has returned, but only 30% of what I used to produce, the milk looks like yoghurt and my beautiful udder is deformed.

Somebody suggested that keeper ring a homeopathic vet, which he did. But he didn't want to pay for a call out because he wasn't sure that prescribing little balls of sugar was worth the cost.

The vet did his best over the phone, but Belladonna and Pulsatilla didn't make any difference to my problems.

My keeper then luckily decided to invite the homeopathic vet to our farm.

He told the following about me: "From a young age, she has been very easy to handle. She had a severe passage of coccidiosis with severe bloody diarrhoea, but she recovered very well. When I do her feet, she plays games with me."

He also told the vet that he tried to make me have many calves but the super ovulation effort, with the use of many powerful hormones to collect embryos, produced no results.

During that time the vet sat down in the sun on a bale of straw and observed me while he listened to the farmer. He noticed this unusual horizontal trembling of my eyes that I have always had and nobody had noticed before.

Two symptoms, 6 remedies: inflammation mamma, rolling of eyes:

Belladonna, Bufo, Conium, Chamomilla, Mercurius, Ustilago

Conium seemed indicated (failing of super-ovulation). One 200K dose - no results.

Second attempt: Bufo 30K twice per day for two days and thank you homeopathy; I have become pretty again and can continue to compete with the best of milking cows in Europe. A few months later I produced 14 embryos; they will all become lovely calves.

Bufo is prepared from the toad; a homeopathic kiss brought back the princess.

63) Jealous because I need you. (M Brunson)

Max is the very lively result of a cross between a toy Poodle and a Teckel; it takes 15 minutes for him to stop barking in the consultation room. He is only five but already for many years he has suffered with serious ear eczemas and irritation of the armpits. Over time the skin has become thick and black.

"He is hyper all the time, he is always active, in the car he jumps backwards and forwards, he follows me around everywhere and he is very possessive about me" This is the introductory phrase of Mrs the owner.

The vet notices that, when Max finally calmed down and had taken position on the lap of Mrs, as soon as Mr tried to approach his wife he growled and would bite.

Mrs adds: "What is his is his! I am his goddess. He likes to dominate. He only eats his food if we pretend we are going to take it away. When he whines, he whines, he will go on for hours if we shut him up in a room."

He has had a few misfortunes in the past: an abscess on one of his testicles caused by an insect bite, unilateral oedema of his face and a generalized urticaria following a food poisoning.

"He doesn't like the heat; when the sun is out he will always find a place in the shade. When he is too warm, he wants to be carried.

He follows me around everywhere, he howls if I leave him for a second. As soon as I sit down he sits on my lap. Otherwise he will sleep curled up on Pudding's feet (other dog). He is possessive and difficult."

In the consult room he lies on his back on Mrs' lap facing and examining the vet behind his desk.

"He eats anything but we never see him drink. He hates the sun but he doesn't mind the rain although he doesn't like to be wet. He prefers not too cold and not too warm. He is aggressive to all other dogs, especially big ones; he jumps up at them and tries to bite them. When Pudding is not there he panics and stops eating. He chases cats but only in our garden."

On the impression of the case (jealousy, aggr. sun) Lachesis 30K is given.

Two months later, the owners are really happy: his ears are very much better; nearly cured. But the vet is not happy about what he hears:

He is still agitated, he still barks all the time, he is still possessive, he is still very attached to Pudding. This means that the cure was local. In these cases one knows for sure that the problems will return or something else will go wrong.

New prescription: Lycopodium 30K, no change.

Over the phone two weeks later: Nux vomica 30K. (The author of the prescriptions notes at this point how poor these prescriptions were.)

Third consultation one month later.

Same story, Max is still the hyperactive, controlling and stressed dog as before. His ears are more or less under control. The skin under his elbows is still irritated.

This time the remedy is the right one: Apis 200K. This is followed by an aggravation of the skin, lasting for two weeks. Luckily the owners have been patient during the aggravation. This was probably due to the fact that Max for once started to behave and Mr was allowed to kiss Mrs again after a break of four years.

The ears start to aggravate again three months later together with a breakdown in behaviour. This is all quickly channelled with a new dose of Apis XMK. Two years later Max is still fine.

Apis was selected by using: jealousy, sun aggravates, industrious, no thirst.

It is interesting to note that, a few years ago, Max had a bad reaction to an insect sting and a problem with oedema earlier in his life. These are both complaints associated with this remedy.

The least one can say about Max is that his training wasn't perfect. This doesn't stop a homeopathic remedy from influencing this dog in such a way that he stops taking advantage of the situation and starts to behave more appropriately. Max is still very lively and still very attached to his mistress but the expression of these characteristics is now within normal limits.

64) When I panic, I lose control! (M Brunson)

It is four years of coughing that is the motivation for the consultation of this 18 year old chestnut pony. He started coughing a few months after his arrival in his latest home. "He must have received a cortisone injection before he arrived here" specifies his owner.

"He does well in the winter, unless we put him in his box. When he can keep his head outside he is OK. He starts to cough as soon as spring arrives."

"He is a warm blooded animal; in the beginning there were many difficulties with his companions."
Two observations stand out during the consultation:

- He has an exophthalmia: His eyes seem to bulge out.

- He has this full and energetic way of shaking his head; different from the other horses.

"He is really a slow eater; he empties his manger but it takes him a long time. This is very contrary to his nervous and agitated behaviour; he cannot stand still."

He is OK to examine but is sensitive to pain; small things affect him. He has this fearful look in his eye. Sometimes he seems quite proud.

"One day he spooked and ran off, no way we could stop him. We only found him back the next day in a real state with the remnants of the carriage dangling on his hind legs. It has taken him two months to get over this incident. He was sad and kept his head low."

"He doesn't like being looked at or tickled, when we groom him too long he gets fed up and becomes jumpy"

"We are afraid to let somebody else look after him; when he panics there is no stopping him, he gets anxious and winds himself up until there is no stopping him. He frightens easily from the least thing. He startles easily."

" He is quite intelligent: he is the first horse I have had that will anticipate where we are going and he never makes mistakes. If I make a mistake during competition he always corrects me. He distinguishes very well between competition and leisure."

The contrast between his anxious/nervous behaviour and his slow eating (confirmed by an observation made during the consultation) are very indicative for Aconite. This remedy fits at the same time all other facets of the story. Aconite is even present in the rubric 'clairvoyance'. One dose in the 30K strength solved the cough very rapidly. The remedy was repeated three months later and further news has always been good.

65) I try to dilute my anxiety. (JP Spillbauer)

From the beginning Jazz wasn't trained properly. Being a Jack Russell Terrier, that can always lead to trouble. His troubles came after having been kennelled. He became aggressive to other dogs and people. The owner of the kennel also commented that he went through phases of 'hallucinations'.

At first he was treated conventionally. He received a drug that treats problems of mood and anxiety. The keepers were also advised on retraining. The training program undertaken by the parents of the owner who was treated for depression, proved completely unfeasible.

To make things more complicated, Jazz spend another few weeks in the kennels after one month's 'treatment'.

Then the daughter took over the retraining, with determination and some success. The medication also started to help after two months. Even in the light of these improvements, Jazz is still impossible.

Nearly four months after the beginning of the troubles, Jazz was presented to the homeopath. This was probably his last chance before the owners separated themselves from him.

The person who came to the consultation was well acquainted with homeopathy and delivered this first very important comment about the frantic patient: "He never dreams, compared to my other dogs. He sneezes frequently. Sometimes he claps his teeth in a slow rhythm when he is stressed or something unusual happens.

He doesn't like people coming and going in the house. When he is really agitated he drinks large quantities of water. Twenty minutes later he will reproduce all this fluid in the form of urine! When I have visitors, I take his water bowl away, otherwise I spend the evening mopping the floor.

There you are, that is all there is to say about him."

The observation made during the consultation only confirms what has been said; he has taken up a position behind the glass door of the consult room and barks at the least stimulus.

The owner adds: "He is inquisitive, he wants to find out what happens elsewhere. He has a good appetite. He will stay in his bed as long as nothing new happens. He gets over excited and aggressive as soon as something happens. He goes completely out of control. He is impossible in the car unless we drive on the motorway.

When he drinks his gallon of water when he is excited this only calms him for a short while"

The vet searches for a while in his repertory until he finds a rubric that sounds as follows: Anxiety, drinking cold water ameliorates.

Two remedies: Sulfur and Aconite. Aconite is preferred because of the restlessness and vigilance that characterised this dog.
One 30C dose. He improves.

A new dose in XMK, three weeks later, and the improvement continues. He will receive another dose three months later.

He is then seen again six months later. No further treatment is required. "Over the last eight months he has completely changed, it is incredible; it is as if he has a completely different character."

Jazz doesn't fight with other dogs anymore, he drinks normally, he is not anxious anymore and he has started dreaming again; he has become normal.

In the summer he spend 14 days in the kennels without any problems.

66) A lucky winter break? (M Brunson)

On a winter Saturday a good friend and colleague rings to ask whether he could drop in a two months old puppy that has been hospitalised three days earlier and that needs further intensive treatment for severe diarrhoea. He is due to leave on holiday. His locum will take back the case when she arrives on Monday.

He tells the poor animal's story: "Nicky was purchased ten days ago in a non-reputable pet shop by a girl as a present for her mum. Two days later I saw the puppy because she was coughing her lungs out. She received antibiotics and a cough mixture and two days later hemorrhagic diarrhoea started. She received stronger antibiotics and intestine capsules but the next day I had to put her on a drip because she had started vomiting and was dehydrated."

As a service to a friend, the vet accepts. His colleague comes in the evening and installs the puppy in one of his kennels in his absence.

The next morning the homeopathic vet finds himself in front of the poorest looking puppy in the world. She is skin and bones and has the saddest look about her. He grabs the sheet with instructions for various injections, pills and re-hydration mixtures that his colleague left him and tries to force the first pill down her throat. Nicky fights the treatment with all the strength she has left. After many attempts, the pill disappears down her throat.

He then draws up two small and one bigger syringe of medicine and starts to feel like a brute, forcing such terrible treatment onto this poor little creature that is just getting worse despite all the medicine she is receiving. His mind is haunted by the story of this poor puppy transported to the shop, then to the new owners, then to the vet and then to a different vet; he hesitates to give the three injections.

At that moment, a sign of nausea and the pill that went down after much struggling comes up accompanied by a large amount of liquid.

He drops his syringes and thinks by himself: if she is going to die she might as well die being treated mildly with homeopathic medicines. He throws all the allopathic drugs in the bin; the pup will stay here until cured or die!

The whole family gets involved: wife and three daughters. Everybody spends some time to observe the puppy in order to collect as many symptoms as possible.

She puts herself in a corner against a radiator. The stools are nearly pure blood; nothing but liquid. She breathes heavily. She is like a little skeleton. She is calm and looks sad. She doesn't want to drink or eat. Indifference to everything, even their presence. She sighs when they stroke her. Both nostrils are blocked with dry crusts. She only gets up when she needs to pass her stool. Urine is dark brown.

First prescription, Sunday afternoon: Pulsatilla 30K followed by a 200k in the evening.
Next morning, she is still alive but produced two very liquid stools. She needs a different remedy!

Mag-c. on the symptom of marasmus and 'abandoned child'. Not much change. She tries to cough but is too weak to cough.

New prescription in the evening: using stool forcible and bile in urine.

Crotalus horridus is given in 30K several times in the evening.

The next morning she is still alive and consents to drink a few drops of water. The whole family agrees that she is looking a bit better but it is still difficult to say in what way. While they discuss this in front of her cage they notice that she doesn't has the strength any more to sit up; her two front legs slide apart when she makes an effort. She has no muscles left. Nobody wants to make a comment, is she going to make it?

She receives four further doses during the day.

Wednesday morning her breathing is better; she makes no effort to cough any more. She has drunk several times and has stopped vomiting. Is she really improving? Crot-h. several times during the day.

Thursday: stools have become like thick sauce and she has changed places several times. When we arrive close to her kennel she gets up to greet us. The remedy is continued several times during the day.

The next day a little food is forced into the mouth and she retains it! No treatment but she is still very weak and there is still some blood in the urine.

Saturday: nobody in the family dares to talk about her. There is no improvement. Is she going to make it? There are again many hesitant thoughts in the vet's mind. Am I on the right remedy? Should I look for a different remedy?

Same remedy but in 200K, once.

Sunday: she sniffs at some food we present but we still have to force it down. She follows us around now; it looks like she is going to live! Another dose of Crot-h 200K.

His friend has come back from holiday. The case is discussed and it is decided that she will stay where she is.

Monday: She walks more steadily. When we arrive, she lies on her side and lifts her leg so we can tickle her belly. Stools are still liquid but some matter has appeared in it. She also eats her first teaspoon of dog food.

Tuesday she starts to play with the young kitten that has been investigating what the whole family was doing in the hospitalisation room every day. She eats well now.

The next day it is the 31st December; she goes home; a nice day to end the year. The whole family is a little sad to see her go home. It is as if Nicky was glad the conventional vet had gone on holiday.

Epilogue:

Nicky is seen again eight years later. She has had no problems during her life. She has suffered with eczema for a few months. Conventional treatment hasn't been satisfactory and she arrives in the consultation room of the homeopathic vet who had saved her life so many years ago.

The consultation does not bring anything really useful to indicate one or another remedy. The vet then gives her a dose of Crot-h. 200K just as when she was ill as a puppy. The eczema disappeared in a few days!

67) I like the children but I am jealous of them. (A Dubois)

Odin is a real Groenendael dog: he is nervous, bites vets, loves children and hates the neighbour. He has very itchy calluses on his elbows and hocks. He received steroids and antibiotics without any success. Somebody even gave him a dose of Calc-c. MK!
He is really lovely: he steals food from the table, he is startled by noise, he is jealous of the children although he really likes them.

He eats very rapidly, and salivates all the time; even when he sleeps. He is stubborn and hates to stay alone at home.

A short but powerful anamnesis.

Salivation at night, jealousy and desire for company alone aggravates, points towards Mercurius sol. This remedy is also present in itching eruption on elbow and hands.

He receives a 200K dose.

Two months later there is still some itching on the left elbow. One dose in 200K.

There is a reoccurrence of itching ten months later: one 200K dose. Then an MK dose is necessary one month later to finish off a few symptoms that are left and that is the end of Odin's skin problems for several years.

68) Again injury but no Arnica. (M Brunson)

This five year old cross breed bitch is normally rather aggressive: she always barks at everybody that comes close to her. When she is brought in the surgery she had had a car accident ten days prior.

Contrary to her usual self she accepts all treatment that is administered "as if she waits for us to help her".

She has multiple superficial lacerations worse on her hind legs: they are swollen with oedema. She has a temperature and drinks less then usual and only wants cold drinks. Her nose and two front paws are cold. She likes to lie against the wall.

Arnica? Well no: mildness, no thirst during fever, cold hands, cold drinks desire, constitutional effects of wounds.

Three doses of Pulsatilla 30K over 36 hours and without the need for antibiotics or painkillers she returns to good health in two days. The wounds heal in no time.

69) I need some encouraging but when I get going there is no stopping. (M Brunson)

"Roscoe eats stones! None of my other dogs do this."
Roscoe is a five months old Siberian Husky, specially imported from Canada to improve the lines in a breeding kennel.

"He is the calmest dog I ever had, he is happy everywhere. He is the puppy that takes the most effort to start playing. On the contrary he talks and whines all the time to express his disapproval when I take him in my arms or for a walk.

He is a gourmand and independent. The bitches that are only three weeks older than him molest him; he doesn't react, he is too nice, he accepts domination. He is a softy, he has no personality. His mum died of an acute form of cancer of the liver a month ago at the age of six.

Roscoe is only interested in eating. He is always chewing something. Sometimes I feel like shaking him to tell him to do something; to react!"

A dose of Calc-c. 30K stops the stone eating but doesn't help the pup with his inner problem.

Three years later, Roscoe is presented with serious locomotors problems. "It started after a training session in the snow. He is stiff, after a few hundred yards he improves but he is still not right on the left side and lacks in dynamism. He is still the quiet and calm dog he was before. He has never been in any mischief in his life.

I always need to incite him to do something; he is too calm. He talks to me when something is not right. He talks to me all the time. For a fortnight he has been glued to my feet and growls when the others come close. He feels the cold at the moment and prefers to be rolled in a duvet (unusual for a S. Husky).

Yesterday after a short walk he was completely tired. He is worse coming down a hill. When he has to stand up too long he leans against something. A year ago he was treated for uremia and itching. He is always hungry and has a slow pulse. His eyes are losing their spark and his coat is becoming dull.

I separated him from the female with whom he shared his box, he didn't mind. He is startled by noise."

Lachesis on the base of jealousy, loquacity: bad choice; no result.

Result from a blood sample: urea is OK but there is a high level of eosinophils in the white blood cell count.

He receives Mezereum (Myositis suspected from high eosiniphil count and 'slowness') in 200K potency. He improves rapidly for a few days and then relapses.

"He cuts all contact with the other dogs of the pack and does not interact with them, until three bitches come on heat; he comes back to life but stops eating for a week. (Even in the consultation room the vet has to push him back several times when he falls in love with his legs). His gait is still unsteady.

He lost weight and has become as lean as he used to be at the age of six months. He is dependant upon me and growls when the others approach. He looks for my encouragement to start eating or to make an effort. He likes physical contact; it appeases him.

When we go out on a walk he will be in front. He doesn't come back to me; if he has gone too far he will sit and wait for us to join up. At the end of the walk he wants to go faster and faster; we can't go fast enough."

Calcarea phos. 200K. one dose: he improves a little but not enough to justify further use of the remedy.

A month later he receives Phosphorus 200K: no change.

He then receives Rhododendron 30K, which helps him somewhat but still no real homeopathic improvement.

New consultation: "He is lacking in energy, his ears are cold. He takes longer than the others to wake up, he needs lots of encouraging. He takes small steps when he walks. He doesn't like to be brushed or touched; when a fly approaches him he shivers. When I am with him, he snarls at the other dogs and will bite"

He receives Causticum 200K: no change.

On a quiet evening the vet picks up his file and asks himself what is really homeopathic in this case?
He needs encouraging to do things
When going for a walk, at the end he can't go fast enough!
He talks a lot; communicates with the owner.

The remedy that has this in its nucleus is Taraxacum. One 200K dose and finally there is a homeopathic reaction. He will take the remedy two more times in four months and becomes better than he has ever been before. He no longer needs any encouragement and engages normally with his friends of the pack. He is still a little slow to start but he gets going without the need to push him. He joins in play activity all by himself.

Taraxacum is what is generally referred to as a small remedy. This usually means that this remedy is not well known in the homeopathic world and therefore not often used. (And probably not well known because not frequently used)

It is often the Owner's determination combined with the effort and honesty of the homeopath that allows for successful prescription in such cases.

This case also reminds us that it is necessary to find what is peculiar in the patient to be successful. Selecting remedies based on their remedy picture does not always work that well.

70) I am not sure. (D Notre-Dame)

When, after many months of various treatments for Prosper's chronic and progressive skin problems, a diagnosis of Discoid Lupus Erytrematus is made, the prognosis is steroids and antibiotics for life.

Prosper is only 18 months old! The future looks bleak and he has lost already five kilograms. His sister has also just been diagnosed with the same disease; his reputed Labrador origins don't seem to warrant a quality life.

When he arrives at the homeopath's consultation he is loaded with antibiotics and steroids.

"He is lethargic, mild and affectionate. He is very kind but he defends himself against the other dogs; he stands his ground. He will only play with his sister, I think he is bored.

He had a problem on his shoulder that disappeared after the use of a homeopathic complex. He is friendly with everybody.

He is not stupid but he is slow in showing his affection; it will take some time for him to come up to me when I call him.

He is always hungry. He drinks normally and his stools are OK.

He still urinates like a puppy, he is timid but he starts to show some assurance. He is not interested in bitches. He gets tired during his walks; he stops and refuses to continue. He limps regularly.

In the night he often gets up to change places. If he wants to go out he makes a tiny noise. He rubs his ears against the bed. He doesn't mind being on his own."

Regardless of his weight loss, he is still overweight. His heart is slow and he moves slowly. He has several lipomas and his nose is cracked.

Based on his slowness, obesity and skin aspect and mostly his irresolution, Graphites 200K is administered.

Two days later his owner rings in to say how he has changed; he recovered his dynamism and the skin already started to improve.

One month later he has a normal body condition and his skin is completely healed. Only his nose and pads are still dry.
A further MK dose takes care of these last details and Prosper starts a new life without problems.

71) Gas cramps. (M Brunson)

Emergencies are rare in this vet's practice but when one of his regular farm clients rang for once he sounded concerned. He would normally joke and say that he has a dying animal but the calf for which he rang up one morning was really unwell.

Twenty minute later the vet was on the farm. A three month old calf lies in the middle of the stable. Suddenly he jumps up and starts to kick in all directions, he calms down for a minute and then starts all over again. He is very violent and vet and farmer are worried he might break a leg. The whole session ends five minutes later with the calf stuck in the fencing of the stable.

The problems started one hour ago just after his evening meal.

The vet attempts to take his temperature; the calf resists this with normal calf behaviour; he wiggles a little but doesn't fight this intrusion with the same energy with which he expressed his abdominal cramps.

While the thermometer sits in the anus to measure the temperature, the vet is blessed with a continuous flow of gas and loose stools over the thermometer and his hands. The calf's abdomen is slightly bloated. His temperature is 40º C (1.5 degrees too high).

Just after the temperature measurement, the vet had the impression that a larger evacuation of gas seemed to appease the calf.

The following symptoms are used for repertorisation:

Restless from pain, pain in abdomen after eating, violent pain, paroxysms with pain, obstructed flatulence.

This produces the following remedies: Colocynthis, Arsenicum album, Chamomilla, Plumbum, Belladonna, Kali carb.

The farmer is left with three vials: one with Coloc. 30K, one with Cham. 30K and one with Plumbum 30K.

The instructions are to start with the first vial, a few drops every 20 minutes, if there is no improvement after 2 hours, he should use the second vial in the same way and then the third if the second remedy didn't help.

The next day the farmer rang back to say that after 2 administrations of the first remedy all had settled and the calf was eating normally that morning.

This is a much better system of using several remedies in case of doubt. It is always more efficient to give them one after another than all of them together. With this system, it is possible to stay in control of the case.

72) I am so deaf that I cannot see. (M Brunson)

On a Saturday morning, Mrs C walks in with Kim her poodle cross. He finds it difficult to keep his balance and walks like a drunk. He walks straight into the wall. A few minutes later it is obvious he can see because he navigates normally around the legs of the table. "He seems deaf" says the owner.

His pupils are dilated, his temperature is slightly below normal. "When he lifts up his leg to urinate he falls over, he drops with his face in his dish when he eats. Over the last few days his head has wobbled from left to right like a puppet. It all started seven days ago after he received an injection for his ear problems. Four days ago he had bad indigestion."

"He is full of arthritis. All his joints crack. He regularly has ear infections. This happens three to four times per year; he then receives an injection of steroids which stops it each time."

The obvious remedy in this case is Helleborus. A 30K dose three times during the day, and in the evening he is already better. This improvement continued without further treatment. No repertorisation was made; the comments of the owner that he seemed deaf when it looked in the consultation room that he was blind was a strong indication for this remedy. The wobbling movement of the head was another (The Helleborus patient says 'no'). Helleborus is also present in ailments from suppression of skin problems (otitis).

73) Fever? No: hypothermia. (M Brunson)

This little queen has been unwell since the morning. She has also lost her balance: when placed on the floor, she rolls over on to her back, gets up again, turns around in a circle for a while and then runs to the side of the room and hides behind the radiator.
"Since she has been unwell, she has been hiding under the blankets of my bed."
Her pupils are dilated and her temperature is below normal. Her pupils don't respond to light.

Hiding herself
Vertigo, turning in a circle
Dilated pupils, insensible to light

Belladonna, one 200K dose and the next day she is fine again. It is interesting to see that even in cases of hypothermia, Belladonna reputed for its activity in fevers can be indicated.

74) Visions of terror. (B Heude)

Soolie has the most loving owner who gives her the best of care and never stops wondering what could go wrong. Soolie lives with Isis, also a Shi-tzu bitch, in an apartment in the middle of a busy town.

At the age of seven she is presented for lumbar pains and fear of lorries and bikes.

"Soolie is a cheerless dog; she doesn't play. She will stay the whole day on the sofa without even making the effort to come up to me for a cuddle. She is not affectionate anyway. But when we go for a walk, she will stop for every person we pass to be stroked!

She likes to go on a walk provided the walk is not too long. She doesn't want to come on the balcony of the apartment because she fears the noises of the lorries and bikes. If the window of the balcony is open, she will hide away in the bathroom because of the noise. This is very strange because when we walk in the street she is not afraid of the noises.

She is very calm, she never barks; she is always asleep.

When we go down with the elevator, she whines; the elevator does not go fast enough for her; she wants to be in the street to meet people and be fussed.

In the house she will accept stroking by my friends but not for long. She will put herself in a calm corner of the house. She doesn't like it when there is too much noise.

She hates the warm weather; in the summer she wants to be showered with cold water. She is happy in the winter but she doesn't like to walk in puddles and prefers the comfort of the inside temperature; she never lies against the radiator.

She doesn't like it when the rooms are too light; she goes through them with her head down.

Her appetite is irregular. She is not very interested in her food but she could eat processed sausages every day.

When her back aches, she moves around and makes little complaining noises. When the pains come up at night, she goes and lies on the carpet in the bathroom; the same spot where she goes when she flees from the noise. It is the calmest place in the apartment.

Sensitivity to noise and light, love for all the people in the street and back pain suggest Phosphorus.

One 200K dose.

One month later: the pains have disappeared but they came back when she got frightened by a demonstration in the street.

One dose Phosphorus MK.

The back pain goes away again.

When the back pain reappears again two months later, the owner successfully treats this episode with a dose of aspirin.

One month later: She is not well. She is sad, there are no more back pains but her fears got worse.

"She looks ill, the people in the street must think that I don't look after her. Sometimes she finds it difficult to get up. She will walk to her dish, sniff and then walk off again.

She hides in the darkest place of the apartment when a lorry goes by. She used to take herself to the bathroom but now she hides in a dark place behind the radiator. She has also become fearful in the street; she is startled when a door shuts."

Phosphorus may have solved the back problems but the remedy has not stopped Soolie from getting worse. The remedy had no homeopathic action; another remedy is needed.

Desire to hide in a dark corner, feigning disease, fear of strangers, fear of noise and light indicate Belladonna.

One 200K dose will very rapidly bring Soolie to normal behaviour. In three weeks time, she becomes lively and stops minding the noises from the street. She still likes to be fussed by passers-by, but to her great satisfaction, her owner now also gets the attention. Of course there are no more signs of or talk about back pains.

This is a nice example about how remedies are efficient in different case situations. Such examples are there to confirm that it is best not to decide too quickly on the remedy for the patient, but to take the time for holistic case taking independent of the diagnosis of the patient.

75) Dull fear. (B Heude)

It is only at the age of five months that Black, a Weimarer dog, was allowed to join his new family. He was the smallest and the most frightened pup in the litter. It took him much longer then his littermates to become fully grown enough to move in with his future owners.

Very early in his life he develops a staphylococcus skin infection on his feet, chin, nose and lips.

The first consult lasts 1.5 hrs. and reveals very little homeopathic information. Black is affectionate, nice, a good gun dog, patient. "He is always with us, he always wants to sit on our laps. He sleeps against us on the bed. He is afraid when he is on his own. He sleeps most of the time, he stays in bed until 11 a.m."

He receives: Phosphorus XM based on his mildness and sleepiness until 11 am

Two months later in March: "I have the impression he is better, he gets up earlier in the morning, sometimes even at 7 am."

The lesions on the nose and front paws are healed. No prescription.

May: Black comes in because there he has a severe outbreak of skin infection. "He eats less, he stays in bed until 11 again."

Vet: 'In what way is Black different from other dogs?'

"From the beginning, I noticed that he sometimes falls asleep while standing; this happens when I prepare his food. He just wakes up in time not to fall over. It gives him a stupid look.

He is afraid to go in the cellar and he doesn't want to go in lifts. He goes in the water until his belly reaches the surface. He wants to feel the ground because he does not have the instinct to lift his head out of the water to breathe. When he was young, he was afraid of his reflection when he walked by a mirror. He barks at his shadow in the dark.

He doesn't digest carrots, we can see them in his droppings."

Based on all the fears and his growing problem as a puppy, Calc carb. MK is prescribed.

June: Following the remedy the skin got really bad followed by an improvement two weeks later.

"When the skin was at its worse, he scratched a hole in a door because we left him on his own. If he hasn't got his bed, he is lost and sleeps standing."

As usual, during the consult, Black is standing behind his owner, his eyelids droopy with a sleepy expression.

No prescription.

End June; he has improved: most skin lesions have disappeared and he is much better in himself, more alert. He still doesn't want to go down into the cellar.

Calc-c. XMK in an effort to obtain further progress.

This prescription wasn't very helpful; the vet comments here that he hasn't taken the time to sit down long enough during the last consultation. The so-called improvement may have been more wishful thinking than real. The skin was better, but inside himself Black had not found peace yet. As a consequence, three months later, a very severe subcutaneous infection of his left front leg broke out.

Black is put on to antibiotics for fear of blood poisoning.

Several homeopathic consultations between September and June the next year.

The skin lesions come and go, Black is still the sleepy dog he used to be. "He is like a baby, when he is with me in the garden he is stupid; he doesn't know what to do. He is still lost when he hasn't got his bed to sleep on."

Pulsatilla, Arsenicum album and Silicea do not make any difference.

August: new consult, no new information.

The vet decides to use what he observes and what is constantly present: he has a stupid expression (his owner does not agree), he has no ideas, he falls asleep, he is like a baby;
Three remedies: Hyosciamus, Nux moschata, Opium
Opium 15C is administered once.

Things go very quickly from here: Black changes, he becomes much more active.
One month later he receives a 30C dose because some of his previous symptoms still show up from time to time. He still has his skin problems but they don't cause him any discomfort anymore.

October: he is like a puppy again or, lets say, for the first time. Nearly all his skin lesions have disappeared. He has no more fears.

Seven months later, he comes in to be vaccinated. He is very well but his owner has noticed that over the last few weeks his stools have become dry. She fears a relapse of his problems
A new dose of Opium, XMK this time.

The case is published four years after this episode; Black has never been ill in the meantime.

It pays to be patient in homeopathy!

76) Two diseases, one remedy. (B Heude)

Frou-frou is a cross-breed queen who lives peacefully with three other cats in the comfortable house of their owners. She is three years old when her problems start.

When finally the owners decide to go for homeopathy, she has been treated unsuccessfully during six months for recurring diarrhoea and periods of anorexia. When she is unwell, her abdomen becomes large and painful from accumulated gas. The diarrhoea is yellow and mushy, she also vomits during these episodes.

Her owner does not add much to the case: "She has no fear, she is mild, she sleeps against me during the night. Sometimes, she chases the other cats off the bed. At the beginning of the evening she will come under the covers; then she becomes too warm and sleeps above the covers."

Vet: talk to me about her food: "She loves eating, she eats very rapidly. Once finished, she goes and finishes the bowls of the other cats. She never drinks milk, but if we eat an ice cream, she will jump up on the table to get her part. She loves fat; she will eat the fat of a piece of ham and leave the meat."

The digestive signs and alimentary preferences indicate Natrum sulfuricum.

She receives one 15C dose.

Her problems stop very rapidly and she is fine for three years.

Then there is an outbreak of infectious ringworm in the cat family. Frou-frou is the last to develop the typical skin lesions. She has several around her head.

The vet asks for any further information to add to the file he has on Frou-frou.

"She is authoritarian. She will punish the other cats if they don't behave; she bites their ears. Everything has to go as it should"

This confirms the remedy she previously received: one dose Nat sulf. 15C.

Three weeks later all the fur has grown back. (without the use of anti-fungal treatments).

Three years later she is still fine. She stayed in control of the cat family but stopped biting their ears - homeopathy is a kind medicine.

77) What a smell! (A. Blanchy)

Diane used to be a very pretty brindle boxer; when she comes to the surgery one April day she is very thin and looks dreadful.

Four months earlier, she was rushed into the local vet's hospital when she caught a stick in the back of her throat: general anaesthetic, removal of the pieces of wood, thorough clean out and antibiotics.

The wounds in the mouth heal very well but after a week, Diane is not right. Antibiotics are stopped for a while. This makes no difference and her temperature starts to rise. An ultrasound of the neck is carried out in search of a piece of wood that may still be lodged in the back of the throat. Nothing is found and Diana is put on antibiotics again.

A month later two fistulae appear under the neck. They discharge a smelly thick liquid containing a few traces of blood. Explorative surgery is carried out, no more pieces of wood are found. More antibiotics. A month later another ultrasound examination is carried out but nothing is found.

Diane is still very unwell and receives continuous antibiotics. A second surgery is carried out, again without results.

The owner then finally decides it is time to visit a homeopath.

Diane is very thin, sad and from her neck discharges a fetid very smelly liquid, noticeable from a distance. As soon as she walks into the surgery, it is like death has arrived.

Based on the suspicion of the presence of a foreign body and the awful smell of the discharge from the two fistulae, Pyrogenium 200K one dose is administered.

The following day, during the afternoon walk, Diana suddenly starts to cough and expectorates a piece of wood the size of a finger. She continues her walk as if nothing has happened. The next day the two fistulae are closed over and when she is seen again one week later at the surgery, they are hardly distinguishable and Diana has regained weight and her energy.

Homeopathy, a slow medicine?

78) I hate you, I will kill you! (A Dubois)

Macintosh is normally a charming 9 year old Yorkshire terrier. He is brought to the surgery to be put down.

The owners are worried because he goes mad when their grandchild comes to stay with them; he gets angry and throws himself at the baby-car and shreds the wheels. "If we let him he would kill the baby!"

Macintosh had previously been treated successfully with Natrum mur. MK for depression when the owner's daughter got married. He was very close to her.

The same remedy is not repeated in this case: the dilution of previous prescription was high enough to warrant a long acting effect; Macintosh should not develop such dreadful behaviour. Natrum muriaticum was therefore just a partial remedy.

Jealousy with rage, driving to kill or crime and bites everybody who disturbs him: Hyosciamus MK.

It takes a week for Macintosh to calm down and accept the baby.
Then another problem occurs...
A few months later the owners come with him to the surgery for a vaccination. They ask whether the vet has a little powder to stop Macintosh from licking the baby. He has not only accepted the baby but had started to protect him. He has become so fond of the baby that it is difficult to stop him from licking the baby all the time. The baby's father is complaining; he is a maniac on cleanliness; he takes three showers per day... .

79) Geriatrics or paediatrics? (A Dubois)

At the age of twelve, Elan has a very lovely life: he goes for walks every day with his retired owners and plays quiet ball games with them in the garden. Every time he feels like having a game, he comes up to them with his ball and they have a good time together. When he wants to go for a walk he comes to them with his lead. Elan is well trained and sleeps quietly downstairs until one day.

At the end of November he started to wake up in the middle of the night, at twelve or one o'clock to enter his owners' bedroom with his ball or his lead in his mouth; he wants to play or go for a walk and wakes them up by tapping them with his paw!

This happens now every night. To be able to sleep, they have to give him sleeping pills or tranquillisers. Elan looks awful since he received these drugs. As soon as they are stopped, he is back at the side of the bed ready for a game or a walk, at the wrong hour.

There is a remedy that is well known in children for this kind of behaviour: Cypripedium pubensces.

One 200K dose and 48hrs later the owners can enjoy normal nights again.

Two years later, Elan relapses. A new dose of the same remedy solves the problem again in two days.

80) Closed in his little environment and intolerant to warmth. (B Heude)

It takes a few years before the owners of Tom, a Tibetan Terrier, finally turn to homeopathy in trying to solve the chronic lameness of their dog. Already at the age of six months X-rays showed the presence of arthritic change in both hips. Over the years, the pain has been more or less controlled with oligo-element treatments.

At the age of six the progression of the disease is confirmed with a new X-ray: the sacral vertebra have become involved in the disease process. The possibility of future paralysis hangs like a sword over his head. This would be a disaster as his owners are enthusiastic ramblers. Nevertheless, after having proposed homeopathic treatment several times over all those years, it is still not an option for these clients; further oligotherapy and painkillers are prescribed when required.

Two years later, things are considerably worse; he doesn't want to be groomed anymore. He becomes aggressive when his owners want to dry his hind legs. Behaviour therapy improves the problem.

When finally, at the age of ten, he has his first homeopathic consult, he cannot get up the stairs anymore.

"Apart from his hip problems, he is never ill. He is the healthiest dog. He has never really liked to play: he will run after the ball twice and then loses interest.

He has no fears. He doesn't like the heat; he prefers the cold. He eats everything and digests everything. He sleeps a lot and snores."

What are his good and bad sides?

"He is stubborn, he comes to us when he decides to. He doesn't go up to people to greet them; he doesn't need their sympathy unless they give him something to eat. He wants to be stroked only by us."

How is he with the other dog?

"Tom is dominant; although he arrived after our other dog and is six months younger than him."

What else?

"His breeder said he was the most gourmand and stubborn of the litter"

What else?

"He is very quick when there is food about or when he hears animal noises on the television."

What affects him most?

"As long as he is with us, everything is fine for him."

What is the most surprising thing about him?

"We can interrupt him at any time, he will lift his head and then put it down again; he has a simple life: he eats, he sleeps and only gets up for his walks. The rest of the time he follows us around in the house."

He receives one dose of Sulfur 200K. This prescription is made based on the atmosphere of the consultation. He is quiet, rather lazy, only thinks about food and doesn't care about other people.

The remedy worked quite well: in a few weeks all signs of lameness are gone.

Four months later during a vaccination consultation, the results are judged very satisfying: Tom doesn't limp. He is still the same: not interested in other people; his owners are enough for him. He is still a charmer with the bitches.

Six months later, his owners are worried: his back cracks when they lift him. The cracking noise is really impressive when he is examined. X-rays show an aggravation of the arthritic lesions of the spine.

Sulfur was not a perfect remedy: it stopped his pains but hadn't stopped the progression of the disease. It is very necessary to find a different remedy.

A new consultation brings further information.

"He is aggressive when we annoy him; when we brush or wash him. He shows his teeth. He loves being fussed and can't get enough.

He loves swimming in a lake up in the mountains where we often go for a walk (very cold water). He knows what he wants. He has his tranquil life. He is slow for everything apart from his food, walks and when he hears animals on television. He is awkward sometimes; several times he has run into an obstacle in the middle of the road like a pole or a signboard. The other dog never does this.

He hates the sun. Since he was a puppy he has always refused to lie in the sun."

His desire to have his little life within his closed environment (family, not interested in other people) and his sluggishness towards most things apart from food and television (i.e. things in the house) are very suggestive for Carbo vegetabilis (also loves taking cold baths and likes walking in open air). He receives a 200K dose.

His behaviour worsened for 10 days; he became inapproachable. After that it all settled very quickly and the physical symptoms, the cracking and lameness disappeared.

He was given a new dose one year later, more out of precaution because there was a suspicion that symptoms were coming back.

A year and a half later he received a further maintenance dose. His owners commented that contrary to the other dog, he doesn't seem to get old. He still lives in his quiet world but since his first dose of Carb-v., started playing. Even at his mature age he plays like a puppy when he feels like it.

It is very common to notice that the aging process is very much slowed down for animals that benefit from good homeopathic prescription; they don't just survive their illness but manage to enjoy life in a more efficient manner.

81) I need you but I don't want to be dependant on you. (B Heude)

This is the story of a magnificent black Chow-chow dog of five years. He has a beautiful coat, only because his owner spends hours maintaining it and fighting his regular outbreaks of suppurating skin disease or diarrhoea. The owner works in a homeopathic pharmacy and already used all the homeopathic remedies that are indicated for these conditions according to popular self-medicate homeopathy handbooks. The successes have never been lasting.

On clinical examination, the rest of a healing hot spot (circular infectious skin disease aggravated by licking and biting) is found on his right hind side. He has also a lick granuloma on his left fore leg. His owner describes his regular yellow diarrhoea outbreaks: they are the signs of reoccurring colitis.

All three symptoms can be associated with a degree of continuous anxiety state that shows through physical symptoms.

"He has one to several diarrhoea attacks per month, they don't affect him. His skin troubles only break out when we are not there. When the skin heals, the diarrhoea comes back.

He is chilly; he doesn't like the cold or the wet. He hates to be wet, even in the summer.

He is not sociable; neither with people nor with dogs. When he doesn't know them, he growls, when he does know them he sticks to them like glue.

His skin problems always start when we come back from weekend or holidays. He stays with my parents when we are away and is OK with them. When we go back to work and leave him alone at home he bites himself raw and the skin problems start.

As soon as one of us gets up he follows that person around. He always has to see us; he will sit in the middle of the house to check where we are.

He is a quiet dog who lives for his habits; he is very worried when we change them. He doesn't want to be disturbed; he doesn't like it when the television is too loud. Sometimes he opens his mouth to warn us, this is quickly stopped with a tap on his nose.

He is like a cat; he comes and goes as he wishes; he will be at our friend's feet at one moment and then afterwards go off to his bed.

He is slow, things have to rise to his brain before he reacts unless it concerns cheese or walks."

One dose of Abrotanum 200K. (Based on the concept of circular relationship with others)

Gerry is seen again two months later: He does really well. No more skin outbreaks or diarrhoea since last time. This seems to good to be true. The vet asks to find out more in order to assure that this prescription has not just caused a suppression of the symptoms but a real improvement.

"He also stopped vomiting and his lameness got better. (These symptoms were not mentioned during the first consultation) He used to limp when he came down the stairs, mainly when the weather was wet.

232

We gave him a complex of Arnica/Rhus tox/Ruta in these cases. We haven't used this mixture in the last two months.

He is less aggressive with other dogs in the street. The lick-granuloma has also disappeared.

He is dependant and independent at the same time and very obstinate. He is like a cat, we like this; he needs us but when we go for a walk it is as if we are not there because he does his own thing."

A tube of Abrotanum 7C is dispensed to be used for two days in case of lameness.

One month later he is seen by a conventional colleague for acute lameness of the right fore leg. He receives a treatment based on steroids. (It is interesting to see how this treatment will interferes in the further progress of the case. The lameness will reoccur a few times before Gerry's successful remedy controls it again.)

Two weeks after this last episode: Gerry comes in for a vaccination booster. The lameness episode is mentioned. The vet proposes to X-ray the leg. The results show obvious arthritis of the right elbow.

A dose of Abrotanum MK is given one week later. This doesn't stop Gerry from limping several times over two months needing two or three administrations of the same remedy in 7C strength.

Four months later, check up over the phone: no further bowel or skin problems.

Next year during the vaccination booster: he is still doing very well. He is lame from time to time when the weather is wet or when he does too much exercise. The limping goes away without the need for treatment.

He receives one XMK dose. He is off his food the next day and his lameness is very aggravated for 48 hrs. The third day all is back to normal. There is no sign of lameness during the next few months (no painkillers needed regardless of the visible arthritis signs on the X-rays!).

Four months later, he develops diarrhoea when returning home from the parents after a holiday. One XMK dose solves the problem in 24hrs.

Six months later the owners are worried he may fall ill because they are due on holiday for three weeks.

Gerry receives one 30C dose.

The holidays are fantastic and on return all goes perfectly. For more than eight months nobody has seen Gerry limping.

82) Slow but keep going. (B Heude)

Titi is the house cat of an eminent human homeopath; he suffers with chronic gingivitis. He was adopted at the local cat protection centre. He had a special status there because of his pleasantness. He stayed the whole day on the director's desk and very often was allowed to stay at her house; he was the only one that was allowed this special treatment.

The consultation takes place a year after his adoption; Titi is not well because of this gingivitis; his coat is dull. This doesn't stop him from being slightly overweight.

"When I went to the cat protection, Titi seduced me with his looks; did he recognise that I didn't really like cats? His eyes seemed to express all the misery in the world. He walked by himself into the basket we brought to transport the animal we were to take home.

He loves being carried around in our arms. He is always ready to be picked up. He doesn't like fat and develops diarrhoea after drinking milk. He is not very playful; he will stop playing very soon after we attempt to start a game.

He is like a dog; he comes when we call him and follows us when we go for a walk. He goes frantic when the wind picks up before thunderstorms; it is difficult to calm him down; we find it difficult to catch him in these circumstances. As soon as the thunderstorm starts he calms down again.

He doesn't come on the sofa with us by himself; we have to encourage him several times. He is slow in comprehending things. He is slow generally; it takes him some time to react. When I leave in the morning he normally sits at the window to see me out, it very often happens he is not there because he arrives too late at the window!

He wants our approval for everything; it is important for him do well."

He receives one dose of Pulsatilla XMK

He is seen again 18 months later. He still has gingivitis and also developed trembling in his front legs. The remedy had not made much difference.

"He is still slow and he doesn't like us to laugh at this, he will walk off and turn his back on us. If he gets told off, he sits down and pretends as if nothing has happened.

He often sniffs the fresh air that comes under the outside door. He also likes the radiator; he sleeps against it.

He is very loving with people but he defends our garden against all other cats. He is very efficient and quick when a foreigner comes into his garden; he is an agile fighter and could easily play the film part of Bruce Lee."

Based on slowness, storm before and rocking ameliorates, Rhus tox 200K is given.

Two months later, Titi is much livelier than he used to be. "He was subdued for a few days after the remedy but now plays more than he used to. He has lost his fears before the thunderstorm. He is much interested than before; we have problems with the fly syndicate that complains that flies have no peace in our house anymore."

Two years before, Titi was tested positive for FELV (infectious cat virus affecting the white blood cells and glands); this day he tested negative.

He has also lost weight; he regularised his food intake by himself and has a normal body weight now.

No prescription.

Titi receives one MK dose when he is worried about seeing his owners pack before the holidays. When he stays with friends during these holidays, he suffers from claustrophobia; they don't want him to go out because of the danger of the main road close to their house. After a week of complaining, Titi is tied up in the garden on a long lead for several hours per day and is completely happy with this solution!

Over the next eight years, he receives Rhus tox again once when Mrs is absent for several days and he becomes worried. He also started vomiting and seemed ashamed of spoiling the floor.

One 200K dose settles the problem. When Mrs is absent again several months later, there is no problem.

"He still plays like a kitten although he is 13 years old."

Rhus tox, remedy for rheumatisms?

83) A comedian. (JP Spillbauer)

Lucky has not really been very lucky: At twelve he has been treated for 10 years for a fistula on his right hind leg; three surgical interventions over this period didn't make any difference.

He is a nervous German Shepherd. He is agitated and whinges all the time. All these years he never has stopped licking the lesions.

"My husband bought him to have somebody to walk with after his heart attack. It worked out that he didn't really have much time to take care of him because of his illness. It was Lucky who took care of my husband after all.

Once he stayed for a weekend with family he knows and likes when we were away: he vomited the whole time. As soon as he came home it stopped; he showed his disapproval!

When we put an Elizabethan collar on him to stop him from licking, he rubs the wound with the side of the collar.

He sleeps in my bedroom, sometimes he comes up on to the bed."

In the consulting room, regardless of his nervousness, he readily accepts being examined all over. "This is outrageous!" exclaims the owner; "When at home we try to look after his wound he howls when we take off the bandage; what a comedian!

Everyday when we have to change the bandage it is the same pantomime.

He is a charming dog, I don't really like dogs but he is really nice. He is intelligent. He comes with me everywhere and behaves very well. He is anxious; that is why he licks his leg.

What pleases him most is that I do as he wishes. I know I am too weak with him.

When I tell him off, he cowers like a helpless creature; it's pathetic!

He licks his leg all the time, even when he plays with other dogs. Once when we took him on a winter holiday, there was no difference in his licking".

Causticum 30C one dose. (nausea after anxiety, affectionate)

The fistula heals in two months. (After 10 years!)

He needed a new dose six months later and is never ill again until he dies peacefully in his sleep at the age of sixteen.

84) Large toilet problems and a desire to live. (JP Spillbauer)

Indy has suffered with intestinal problems since she was a puppy; she passes enormous stools, is often constipated and has frequent hemorrhagic colitis attacks. She has received as many diagnoses and treatments as she has seen different veterinary surgeons.

She is now five, and none of the treatments have really helped her. She has more and more of the skin allergy and diarrhoea attacks. Alternatively she is often constipated, unable to produce any stools. When she finally goes to the toilet, her droppings are enormous. Her stools have always been rather large.

On examination she has a noticeable amount of stools in her rectum. Her both front legs have irritated skin. She scratches mostly after eating. She receives the best prescription diets available to control her problems without success.

A few times she developed hemorrhagic diarrhoea and needed to be put on a drip twice over the past years.

"She is very playful, she has a great desire to live. She has never been affected by all the interventions and treatments she received.

Two years ago we adopted her mother; she completely dominates Indy.

Indy is very close to me, she is immature, she is my baby. But if somebody dares to annoy me she will defend me ferociously.

She is very clean in spite of her 'toilet' problems. She is very greedy. She thinks about nothing but playing.

When another dog annoys her she bites, she is not as tough as her mother who dominates her.

Her stools have always been much larger than the other dogs.

She is very individualistic, very very individualistic!"

In the rubric 'ineffective urging' one of the remedies is Aloe. The remedy fits the picture of this bitch rather well.

A 200K dose once per day for three days, repeated two weeks later.

Her rectal problems receded by 90% within 3 days after the first treatment, not to come back for at least 18 months (last contact). The skin problems disappeared completely.

85) You touch me I kill you! (L. Van Damme)

It is common to see mares becoming excited when spring triggers the beginning of the breeding season. A little grumpiness, some sensitivity to the legs of the rider, a little bit slower or faster than usual and in some cases very indecent behaviour towards anything that seems male may be acceptable but in this case things got out of hand.

This 15 year old mare had already received numerous treatments (including homeopathic ones) for her behaviour during heat. "She is a nutter when she comes on heat in the spring and it doesn't stop!"

There is not much chance to examine her but just by looking at her you get the picture.

"She doesn't want to take any orders, she doesn't want to be touched and she will rear as soon as you approach her."

She was once transported to a specialist vet; he has diagnosed cystic ovaries like grapes with his ultrasound when she was safely strapped in a strong horse stall.

"She is very difficult to ride; her back becomes hard like wood. She is violent. She is very fast moving. She is afraid of nothing. She is always in a hurry and tries to work well. She attacks other horses. She never stops moving when at work and she hates the whip; she goes tense in the neck and mouth.

She is dominated by the other horses. She doesn't integrate; she doesn't speak to the other horses.

When she jumps the bars, she makes no efforts because she knows the bars will fall off when she touches them. When she jumps a solid fence she pays attention and lifts her legs properly.

She cannot walk calmly into her box; she always rushes in; we have to be careful. Everything she does she does in a hurry.

When she is hurt she doesn't complain.

When she urinates during her heat period, she kicks her legs out like mad. She must be incontinent because she wets herself."

Based on incontinence during heat and the apparent pain when she urinates, Cantharis one 200K dose is given.

To administer the homeopathic remedy she needed a nose twitch.

That was the last time it was necessary to use a twitch on her. Her behaviour improved in two weeks time and the heat periods became normal. There were no more complaints over the next two years.

86) Deprived of everything! (M Brunson)

We stay in the countryside to tell the story of Melanie, a cross-breed dairy cow. She has just had her third calf.

"I have been too severe on the weaning; she had only straw and no water for several days; she hasn't recuperated from it."

Melanie is a very productive milking cow; she had not fully recuperated from her previous lactation period. The severe weaning practice made things worse: she is left emaciated and without any strength. She receives China 30K twice per day for three days, which makes no difference.

The weather turns cold and things get worse: she goes into hypothermia.

A clinical examination a few days later gives no homeopathic clues and the questioning of the farmer gives no further information either.

The vet then tries to imagine what stands out in this case: she is cold, she has been (and still is) hungry, she has been lacking in water.

Based on this observation, she receives Cistus canadensis. This flower (rose) lives in very cold circumstances on rocky slopes where there is only a small amount of earth to plant its roots in: the same circumstances as Melanie: cold, lacking in food and water.

She receives a 30K dose twice per day for three days and very quickly picks up again to normal health.

This is not Paracelse's theory of signatures; it is the application of what is peculiar in the case of the patient compared with what is peculiar about the substance.

87) Spasm from suppression? (E De Beukelaer)

This client has been very patient; it has taken me four years to finally find the remedy for her horse.

The hunting mare started to show symptoms of head-shaking at the age of six. The syndrome had come on rather quickly; a few months after the first signs it became nearly impossible to ride her. As soon as she starts to trot she throws her head around in all directions. The spasms can be felt travelling along her spine. An inexperienced rider would find it very difficult to stay in the saddle. Riding her has become a real struggle and very unpleasant.

The following is the summary of two to three consultations per year over four years.

"She is a very big horse. Since her problems we haven't seen her coming on heat any more. She may show one heat in the beginning of the season (February) and then nothing. We would notice because she is in the field with an old but still very 'motivated' gelding that used to stop eating and sweat for a week when she came on heat.

She is ticklish; she will lift her leg when we touch her belly. She is explosive; she will rear full height when we take her out of the field. One minute later she looks sheepishly as if she doesn't realise what she has done. She is not always considerate and will crush you."

Based on this observation (she is explosive and then seems to excuse herself), she received Glonoine one 200K dose. This remedy stopped the problem within a few days for four months during the summer when it usually presented itself with a maximum intensity. (Previous prescriptions of Belladonna, Bryonia, Kali carb., Aurum-s-n., Cuprum, Natrum mur. did not produce any results)

Then she relapses and further administrations of the same remedy don't make any difference; the remedy was efficient but not homeopathic.

The owner keeps on talking about shocks that go through her back. She is better when the weather is wet. She pushes you around in the stable. Her seasons are absent. On several occasions, a colleague specialist in equine reproduction examines the mare. There is no explanation for the absence of her cycle. Several hormonal treatments fail.

After four years and at least twelve unsuccessful prescriptions, the link between the absence of heat and the appearance of the head shaking becomes clear.

Based on this observation she receives Zincum 200K.

This times she improves slowly. She receives a further MK two months later and an XMK three months later. Over six months time she comes back to normal. All the head-shaking symptoms disappear and she comes on heat again.

The side effect of the prescription is that her old field-companion starts losing weight again each time she comes in heat. He is 25 and cannot really afford these regular weight losses. He is retired somewhere else and our patient is moved to a different place. The latest news three years later is still positive. She competes again at a high level in show jumping.

88) Beautiful eyes. (A Blanchy)

Vodka is a very pretty Siamese queen and 14 years old when she is presented at the consultation. Her owners have been on holiday and she stayed with the parents during this period.

A few days after the return from holiday, something is not right: she stopped eating and walks slowly with her back arched.

The owners refuse antibiotics and steroids; that is OK. They are also not interested in any complementary examinations; that is a little more worrying because no valuable diagnostic and prognosis can be made. Luckily homeopathy can be practised successfully without all this by just using the symptoms of the patient.

The first strange observation is the colour of Vodka's eyes: they are white. This is due to a change of the liquid behind the cornea (in the anterior eye chamber); this liquid has turned milky white. This change has taken place in the few days after the return from holiday.

"She doesn't lie on her side anymore; it is painful for her to lie on her side"
The pain on the right side is confirmed during the clinical examination with a scratch on the vet's hand: when the vet touches the cat's kidneys, she reacts violently in spite of her state of prostration.

For the rest she is a normal Siamese cat; usually she is talkative and follows everybody around in the house. Now she keeps to herself and sits in a corner.

The vet makes a repertorisation using the symptoms that are present: Opacity of vitreous, inflammation kidneys, kidneys pain lying, back pain lying, back pain pressure.

The remedy that is strongest present is Colchicum. One 30K dose brings back her appetite and clears the eyes.

One month later she receives another 30K dose because she hasn't gained her usual liveliness; "she has got older."

There is no news for two years.

Then she is presented again because she has lost her appetite after an abscess broke out. Her eyes have become white again. She receives a dose of Colchicum 30K.

No more news for two years.

Vodka is now over sixteen years old. Her eyes have suddenly become white again and she has developed a vestibular syndrome; she turns around in a circle all the time and doesn't eat anymore.

The owners confirm that previous administrations of the remedy each time had proved successful.

One 200K dose is given. A few hours later she goes to sleep and never wakes up again.

This is another case of euthanasia with homeopathy. There is no information on how ill Vodka really was at this stage because the owners were never interested in complementary examinations. One thing that is sure is that when an animal goes peacefully to sleep after the administration of a homeopathic remedy, it is biologically the time to go. Conventional medicine can in some cases keep the animals going for a while beyond this date. The question is whether they really live their life then?

89) Salt for diarrhoea? (P Froment)

A herd of 130 milking goats suffers from diarrhoea during the month of August. Half of them have been improved with antibiotics. It started after a thunderstorm. Three goats have died.

"Some of them keep their appetite. The diarrhoea starts in the morning. The sick animals are very worn out. They drink large quantities. When we had the same problem two years ago, they died immediately. This year they keep going for a while before they die."

The vet realises that the farmer is feeding too much concentrated food for the amount of milk his goats are producing. This error is put right.

Diarrhoea warm weather, chronic diarrhoea, diarrhoea from farinaceous food, diarrhoea in the morning: Natrum mur. one XMK dose for the whole flock. Within 36 hrs all diarrhoea stops and there are no more casualties.

90) All these adults around me drive me mad. (L. Van Damme)

The vet is called out to see Beau, a 15 year old hunter type horse with skin 'allergy' problems. He lives in big box with view over a pretty garden in a nice yard, has a friendly owner, works only a moderate amount and has friendly mates to roam with in the beautiful fields at their disposal; there is really no reason why he has problems.

"My horse develops small hives on his face and trunk, never on his legs. It usually starts in March or April. This winter he has scratched himself a few times. When he scratches himself, the hives get infected. This happens mostly on his face.

He needs a strong tranquilliser when we clip him. Otherwise he would smash up everything around him.

He only wants to stay in one particular box from where he can see all the other horses, otherwise he wrecks the place. Not any box where he can see the others; it has to be this particular one.

When he has the eruptions on his face, it is impossible to ride him. The skin problem didn't respond to a steroid treatment, it responded to a fungal treatment one year. The next year the same treatment didn't make any difference.

He is rather turned on; one year he mounted a mare several times. At one point we thought he wasn't properly gelded.

He fights with other geldings but when he is saddled he accepts them around him; once he even accepted being bitten on the buttocks without responding.

He is unpredictable: he was happily in a field for weeks with a mare and then suddenly, one day, we found her savaged with bites all over her. This was unexpected, we thought he liked her because he is jealous of her: one day she stood nose to nose over the fence with another gelding, Beau jumped the fence and started battering the other gelding. He even continued when this one was lying on the ground. He can be very violent when he panics.

He likes the calm of the riding school. On several occasions he has bitten people who walked past him. He wind-sucks when there is animosity in the yard.

On the contrary, he never attacks the foal; it is allowed to bite him.

We can't brush his head, he hates sudden movements. He flattens his ears as soon as anybody comes close to him. He is agitated when he is with other horses in the lorry; on his own in the van he is OK.

He is difficult to feed; one day he didn't want to eat his usual food anymore. When we gave it again the next day, he ruined his manger and spilled all the food around. If we change something in his usual ration, the same thing happens. He gets diarrhoea from carrots and molasses.

We don't take him out on hacks anymore; he is a coward. He is afraid of the wind and unusual noises.

He has moods; when he is in a bad mood, it is best not to go in his box because he will kick."

Hatred, aversion company and childish behaviour indicate Cicuta virosa.

245

One 30K dose has solved his skin problems. (Two years feed back). He has also become much more reasonable in his behaviour; it hasn't become perfect but then his owner never really tried to impose herself on him.

91) Stay together. (M Brunson)

Tina is a 10 year old German Shepherd who lives in a kennel in the garden. She comes in the house and goes in the garden in the mornings and evenings. For many years she has been scratching; she has bald patches on the sides. The rest of the fur is of poor quality. Hairs are breaking off and there are little crusts on a greasy skin everywhere. She has crusts on her lips. The skin on the base of the tail is inflamed and painful.

" She eats everything. She barks a lot (the owner considers she is not well trained). She doesn't like the cold; she will bark jumping up and down to keep warm. She guards when it is not necessary (especially when it's cold). She doesn't like potatoes. She is not intelligent. She will bite from behind when she is not afraid; it is as if she needs to convince herself to guard. She does it when we are there.

She always carries something in her mouth.

She doesn't mind the weather; she will sleep outside in the rain. Sometimes she will sleep in her pen. She always sleeps with her head against something. She snores.

She is close to people; she will obey the least request from my youngest daughter. She has searched for a long time for our cat who got killed in a road accident. (She received Natrum muriaticum, which improved her behaviour but not the skin). She eats out of the same dish as the cat. She accepts that the birds eat from her dish.

She has no preferences for any of the members of the family. She got worse when we were on holiday."

The image the story brings to the vet is that of a dog who defends its family and will allow any of them to eat from its plate. She has no preferences in the family. She only defends the property when they are around.

Magnesia muriaticum 30K one dose.

The remedy is repeated twice in 200K over the next year when the skin shows signs of relapsing. Every time the skin settles quickly. Tina is still very sweet but has become more self-assured.

92) The hidden wart that indicated the remedy. (JP Spillbauer)

"Hector has been itchy since we bought him at the age of 2 months."
Hector is now 6 and has been treated with many doses of steroids for a skin disease that has been diagnosed as atopy (allergic skin condition). He is on a special diet and has grown a little belly probably due to the steroids.

His coat is dull, he has moist seborrhoea and still scratches himself from time to time. The scratching often results in a skin infection.

He is a happy dog with lots of energy. He has a dominant tendency towards other dogs. He is good with children and friendly to people. He lives in town during the week and in the countryside over the weekend; this has no influence on his condition."

That is all there is to say about Hector.

After a while, the owner adds: "Six months ago he was operated on for a growth in the middle of his mouth. It has never grown back. Sometimes he has warts on his skin. Two years ago a bee stung him on his lip; it took him one month to get over this. He was really affected by it."

Mouth, warts tongue: seven remedies.

The vet selects Aurum muriaticum based on the reading of the Materia Medica.

One 30K dose has a spectacular result.

Six months later he relapses after having stolen a large piece of meat.

A new dose of the same remedy stops the skin problems in no time.

One and a half years later he is still doing very well.

I cannot think of a better case to show that a prescription is not based on the conventional diagnosis but on what is peculiar in the case!

93) Anxiously restless. (JP Spillbauer)

Tiny is very unclean; she will put her two legs in her litter-tray and then walk off to urinate or defecate anywhere in the house. She is seven and has been scratching herself for four years.

She lives in a house with eight other cats. She is very jealous; if her owners pay attention to one of the other cats she arrives at full speed to request her part of attention.

She needs only two mouthfuls of food per day to keep her weight.

"She is a quiet cat, she never makes any noise but she never sleeps and is certainly not timid: she attacks our Poodle. She never settles down, she keeps on walking all over the place. Doing so she disturbs the others while they sleep. She has to walk and there is anxiety in her expression.

When she stayed with my parents in town, she used to get out of the door as soon as she got the chance. They would find her sitting in the middle of the street or a crowd; she has no fear.

She keeps on attacking the Poodle, it is as if she forgets she.has just attacked him. She has no fear, she lives for the moment.

If we didn't pay attention, she would walk off. She only meows when she wants to get out of a room. As long as she can walk around she is fine."

This seems a beautiful case to find a really nice remedy based on themes and remedy pictures. Well no: over the period of a year she received ten remedies with no success.

Then the vet decides to make an ordinary repertorisation:
Sleepless from anxiety, desire to walk, jealous, aversion food, attempts to escape:
Arsenicum album: three doses in five months and all skin and behaviour problems disappeared.

94) Insecticide and aphrodisiac? (presentation made by a colleague during a study session)

During an outbreak of flu in a cattle herd during the Autumn, even Bill, the proud bull of the herd, is affected. Most of the cows responded well to a classic antibiotic treatment. Bill and a few of the older ladies need some special attention.
Based on the symptoms of the cough, Phosphorus sorts out all the ladies but not the man in the house: he needs a specific prescription.
"He is not very affected by the cough; green-white pus discharges from his nostrils; he is very jealous of his females; we have to be careful although he is not really dangerous. He is very proud; he doesn't like to be handled. Regardless of his temperature he still eats normally. He hasn't lost any weight since he was ill."
Lachesis, Bryonia and Pulsatilla are prescribed one after another with no success. His condition remains OK but his performance with the ladies has gone down. It becomes now urgent to find a cure; he may be made redundant for non-compliance with his job description.

The vet comes down again to have a good look at him. He cannot find much unless – aha! - the bull seems to scratch himself. A closer look reveals the presence of lice; he is covered with them; one would expect him to scratch much more.
Panic in the stable! All the cattle are examined to establish the severity of the infestation - not one louse can be found on them.

249

Skin lice and proud: Staphysagria one 200K dose.

The lice disappear (without the need for insecticides), his cough and nasal discharge clear up and more important: he takes up his job again.

A homeopathic remedy that is at the same time insecticide, antibiotic and aphrodisiac!

95) The showman. (JP Reboul)

This event horse has failed his purchase visit already several times for navicular disease (visible decalcification of the pedal bone on X-rays). He is a beautiful and majestic horse; he puts on the most wonderful performances during competition. This is the reason why several people attempted to buy him but every time their vet failed the horse during the purchase visit.

After examination and discussion with the carer, the only symptom that stands out is that he stumbles quite easily. This happens when he is lead walked. There is not much to base a homeopathic prescription on.

When he is later observed working, there is no sign of hesitation any more; he is a majestic horse; he moves like dream and shows how he enjoys his performance. The stumbling only seems to happen when he stops performing, in between his performances or when he walks from one place to another.

On this notion, the vet prescribes Veratrum album. The remedy is repeated a second time during the event season two months later when a mild sign of lameness is observed.

At the end of the season he is sold and passes a thorough purchase visit with flying colours (no more lesions visible on X-rays).

The buyer of this horse didn't purchase a pig in a poke: when animals improve radiologically it is reasonable to talk of real cure. The future owner has no more chance of encountering problems with this horse than any other. On the contrary, it is likely that because this horse benefited from a good homeopathic prescription he will be healthier than many other horses.

96) If I differentiate, I lose my identity. (S Opolka)

Lassie is a Shepherd cross. At the age of seven she undergoes surgery for infection of the womb. During surgery a large tumour of the right ovary is also removed. Histology reveals a benign tumour.

A week later Lassie doesn't want to eat. Clinically she is fine: no temperature, no inflammation, no pain, no vomiting, nothing.

Homeopathy is needed to help out.

"We have had a cat for two months. Although she chases all cats, she accepted this one because we told her so. She washes the cat, finishes her dish but sits beside her when she is eating. Lassie follows us around everywhere.

She is jealous when we stroke the cat. She is very scared of loud noises and thunderstorms; she tries to hide in the smallest place she can find. I am also afraid of thunderstorms.

If I go away to see my daughter she doesn't eat during my absence. She has been equally sad when my husband was away for a week. She follows him around everywhere. She is very sensitive and exuberant. When she greets our son she talks to him.

She hates chocolate but she loves dainties. She loves apples, she asks for them. She hates it when we play fight; she even defends the cat when we pretend we are going to hit her. She has been very easy to train; she understands everything."

This very close relationship with the family suggests Carcinosinum.

She receives a XMK dose.

251

She started eating again a few hours after having taken the remedy. She has also become more lively and goes out in the garden again which she had stopped doing for a while.

Two years later the owner makes an appointment to remove a mammary tumour. The appointment is delayed because of bad winter weather. The vet suggests giving a new dose of Carsinosinum until the weather clears.

A week later the snow is gone and Lassie comes to the surgery for her operation. The remedy she received the week before has given her new energy, she is less puffy than she used to be. The owner thinks that the tumour has diminished in volume.

An X-ray is taken of her lungs; there is pulmonary invasion in the Right lung. There is also an enlarged lymph node under her right leg.

Surgical intervention is ruled out. It is decided to continue to help Lassie with the remedy that seems to do her so much good.

She receives the remedy again four months later; XMK, because the tumour has ulcerated.

Five months later a new dose XMK because she becomes breathless during her walks. She also started scratching the tumour and a new ulcer starts to form.

Fifteen months later, Lassie is still fine and full of life. The swollen gland under the right fore leg has disappeared. The tumour is still there but hasn't really changed since the beginning (i.e. two years ago).

Do patients always need the removal of a tumour? There are many more cases where tumours have been kept under control or have regressed with homeopathic treatment.

97) Open or closed? (M Brunson)

Until he was 13 years old, Donovan never needed the vet. He lived quietly in the last house of a cul-de-sac with his owner and together they went for long walks everyday. Recently the walks have been reduced because age started to limit Donovan's fitness.

During the month of April, he is presented for coughing. The owners are not interested in homeopathy and he goes home with antibiotics and a cough mixture.

In June, when they are at the seaside, Donovan develops a lung oedema. He is treated in emergency locally. The oedema goes away but his cough gets worse after this.

This time the owners realise the seriousness of his condition and the lack of improvement after various allopathic treatments.

"The cough is worse between 3 and 5 in the morning, he tries to cough up something. After coughing he has a drink. He also coughs every time he gets excited. When he feels the cough arriving he gets up. Sometimes he sneezes after having coughed. When he manages to expectorate, the cough stops. He eats and drinks normally. He doesn't like the rain anymore; he enjoys wearing his coat.

He sleeps against the radiators, he likes the sun. He loves the car; he never coughs in the car. He sleeps on the couch with his four legs in the air. He is not sociable: he barks at all the dogs we come across when we go out with him. He has never done any damage in the house."

Warm stove, cough in old people and expectoration ameliorate; several remedies are present but Causticum is preferred. 12K three times per day for a week. He improves rapidly but two weeks later the cough is back again.

Causticum is repeated in 30K twice.
No result, even worse: four days later he arrives in the surgery with severe respiratory distress; there is an severe lung oedema, especially on the right side. His heart is weak and in severe trouble; he is very lethargic.

In the same repertorisation from previous consultation another remedy appeared which has an indication in lung oedema: Ammonium carbonicum.

He receives a 30K dose every 15 minutes. Three hours later he goes out in the garden to empty his bladder. He even cocks up his leg. The lung oedema has disappeared and the heart sounds happier. Two hours later he jumps in the car when the owners come to collect him.

Over the next six months he receives the same remedy three more times. He continues to enjoy life until he then passes away in his sleep when he is fifteen.

98) When I want it and how I want it. (M Brunson)

"It started when he was six months old on holiday in Spain. A pink swelling appeared under his collar. It spread up to his ear. In eight days it all disappeared with antibiotics. The problems reappeared when we came back from holidays. He has been treated again but this time it took a little longer to disappear. When it came back the third time he didn't respond to treatment any more."

Tell me about him: "George is very nervous. We have been going to dog training for a month; he tends to growl at other males (he is 11 months). Already at the age of three months he tried to growl at us several times. In the club he is considered as difficult."

After 15 minutes, the vet is called out of the consultation room. When he comes back in, George greets him as if he is his best friend.

"During the classes he growled once or twice at the trainer. He learns well and sits at a distance when we ask him to but he doesn't come back when we call him. I am afraid to undo his lead when we walk him, he would run off after wildlife or another dog and not come back. We had to buy an anti-barking collar for him; he used to annoy the neighbours with his continuous yapping. He got the message in a week and goes out without his collar now.

He doesn't like water; he goes around puddles. When he started to dig holes in the garden we disposed of his droppings in them. He quickly understood what we wanted and stopped digging.

When he was young he was very independent, now he is closer to us but if we don't pay any attention to him he goes to his bed.

He is not keen on dried food and we have to change brands all the time. He drinks large amounts but only when the water is fresh. When we have visitors he is more exuberant with them than he is with us when we come back from work.

He is indifferent to the weather. When we approach him he rolls on his back with his legs in the air. We are very fond on him but he is exhausting. He loves playing but what he likes most is going for walks. He is always on the watch out for flies; we don't have any in the house!"

He receives Phosphorus 30K. His neck improves but the problems shift to the eyelids and scrotum.

He comes back a month later and is full of energy: he jumps on the consult table and greets the vet enthusiastically.

"When we refuse him something he goes for his tail and pulls out his fur. Sometimes he behaves like a battered dog; when we call him he is stressed. He likes physical contact; he even lies against us when he chews a bone.

If we want to clean his ears and eyes we have to muzzle him. He is not a big eater; he doesn't finish his dish. When we are on the telephone he pushes up to us to seek our attention. We use a water spray to make him obey; it works but not for long.

He is not a nasty dog; if by accident we tread on his foot he doesn't react and he likes everybody."

Stramonium 30K twice in a day.

Three months later: no improvement.

"George takes a while to learn at the club but once he knows he knows. The most difficult thing is to keep him under control. We cannot really praise him; the least friendly sign from our side and he goes mad again. It is even difficult for him to control himself; when we come home he walks around with a teddy bear in his mouth from excitement instead of greeting us.

He shakes his head for the first five minutes at the start of the walk because he perceives his collar as a constraint."

Crot tiglium and later Lycopodium make no difference.

Thereafter a prescription of Mercurius solves the skin problems. He receives the same remedy five times over the following year and then it becomes clear that the remedy is not really solving all his problems. After a year the skin doesn't respond to this remedy anymore and his behaviour gets worse.

He growls more and more at the husband and the trainers in the club. He becomes more and more attached to Mrs and cries when she is away.

"He is over the moon when visitors come in but he doesn't respond anymore when my husband or sons come home. Although he is very kind to our tetraplegic neighbour he is still difficult to control from time to time. When we walk along the other neighbour's garden he snarls at their Setter; if I pull on the lead he growls at me but doesn't bite. I wonder whether we will ever achieve any results with him. He is full of contradictions he has a worried look on his face.

If he doesn't get what he wants he rubs his face on the floor. He pulls like mad in all directions when he wants to go in a different direction during his walks. He gets more and more self-assured with strange dogs and barks at them but when on two occasions he was attacked he didn't defend himself.

There is one tree he always barks at; we don't know why.

He is not jealous at all, he never asks for any food.

Only the water sprayer stops him. He doesn't like water: when he runs after the ducks he stops dead at the side of the lake.

We can only stroke him when he wants it; after a few minutes he will stop us and go away.

At the club they call him the spoiled brat! We applied all the best advice on dog training, it doesn't seem to work with him."

Intolerant of contradiction, disobedient, capricious appetite, impetuous, capricious:
The remedy in sixth position is Cina:

The notion of discipline difficulties and the fact that he won't understand that he cannot always get what he wants are good indications for this remedy.

One 200K dose spectacularly changes George's attitude: the people at the club wonder what tranquilliser was used on him.

He receives four more doses over the next year for reappearance of a few skin problems. Every time the lesions disappear in no time. His behaviour continues to be 90% better than before.

99) Patience pays. (JP Reboul)

Samba (Oriental cat) is nearly two when he disappears for the first time from his home. When he comes back he is very tired, his little tongue hangs out of his mouth and his balance is unsteady.

The vet prescribes Stramonium 30C over the phone which does the trick. The same remedy works in two more of these 'attacks' he has over the following year.

A year later a new attack of his balance problems appears; this time the remedy doesn't help and he gets worse and worse.

It is time for proper homeopathic reflection.

"He sits prostrated and only comes out of his corner to drink. He drinks more than usual. He eats but not when we bring the food to him; he doesn't seem to recognise his food. It is as if his brain doesn't analyse anymore. He feels cold and sits sometimes with his tongue hanging out of his mouth: his nose dripping and saliva running from his mouth. He has lost his coordination."

On the consultation table he lifts his foot as if to scratch his head. The movement stops halfway and becomes spasmodic like a badly functioning robot.

"One day he had an attack and fell like a dead thing between the bars of the stairs. He is painful on the left side; he swears when we touch his left side."

Automatic motions of upper limbs, protruding tongue, confusion after head injury point towards Helleborus.

Before administrating the remedy the vet reads the Materia Medica of Kent which contains the following observation about the remedy:

"The remedy acts slowly in these slow, stubborn, stupid cases of brain and spinal trouble.
- Sometimes there is no apparent change until the day after the remedy is administered or even the next night, when there comes a sweat, a diarrhoea, or vomiting - a reaction.
- They must not be interfered with no remedy must be given.
- They are signs of reaction.
- If the child has vitality enough to recover, he will now recover.
- If the vomiting is stopped by any remedy that will stop it, the Hellebore will be antidoted.
- Let the vomiting or the diarrhoea or the sweat alone, and it will pass away during the day.
- The child will become warm, and in a few days will return to consciousness - and then what will take place."

The vet warns the owners and the cat receives a 30C dose.

Four days later (after a long weekend) the owner rings to thank for the warning. "Samba is doing really well, but for two days I had to keep convincing my husband not to take him to the emergency service; he vomited several times and developed severe diarrhoea. The third day it all calmed down and two days later our usual kitten was back. He is better than he has been for a year."
He will need the remedy twice more in a year.
Two years later he is still fine.

100) Rather clever. (P Rouchossé)

Husky is a 14 year old pony who has suffered from emphysema from an early age. He used to be a champion show jumper but the last two years it has not been possible to work him properly.

"He is worse when the wind comes from the south, when we use weed killers, when the hay is dusty and when it rains. He becomes sulky when he is ill; he knows he has always been the grand champion in the house; he considers himself superior to the other horses. He imposes himself on them and corners them to show his determination.

He protects the mares. He is cool when he is only with one other horse. When there are more horses around he makes sure that everybody keeps in their right place.

He is intelligent. When he goes to a competition he follows the previous horse in the ring with his eyes to check on the path to follow. He will remember the course and correct any mistakes made by the rider. When it is a timed run he accelerates without asking.

The other day he noticed that the current on the fencing was off and he broke out. When he realised that the current was put on again he made one of the mares approach the fencing to see whether she would jump. He does this every time; when the horses don't jump up he breaks out.

He took pride in his successes, now he is depressed because he cannot compete any more."

Has he any fears?

"A little when we go in the forest but never when he competes. He is not a glutton, he eats normally."

He receives Veratrum album 200K.

He improves for 15 days and then follows a big crisis. Another remedy is needed.

A month later he receives Natrum carb. based on his intelligent behaviour and depression due to his disease.

One 200K dose is followed by a 100% improvement. He goes back to competition and needs a dose three times a year to keep going. Two years later he wins the regional show jumping championship.

101) The image of the origin of the remedy. (B Heude)

Nancy is a little top model Yorkshire terrier who lives with her owner and six other Yorkshire terriers in a nice house. When their mistress goes to work, they all stay at her mother's house.

When she is four, she develops a localised skin infection on her abdomen and neck. A classic antibiotic treatment produces only mediocre results.

A few months later the client agrees to call in help from homeopathy.

"She is attracted by depths. She always lies on the side of a height, the side of the sofa, the side of the steps of the stairs, the back of the car seat. She regularly falls off these high places."

This is verified in the consulting room; placed in the middle of the table she deliberately goes to lay on the side of the table.

"We find her often upstairs on a old balcony where she watches what happens outside through the cracks in the planks. I am worried because the balcony is not safe. She is very curious; she spends hours watching what happens outside through the window in the door. She is the first to find a hole in the fencing to escape to the neighbours. She is very independent; she plays her own games without taking care of the others.

She does everything that is not allowed. When she has a toy, nobody can take it away from her; she is capable of putting a biscuit in front of the others just to annoy them. Not one of them will come closer.

She is calm and fears nothing. She is not aggressive and lets us do to her what we want.

She hates the wind and the rain. She will pretend she limps if I want to take them out in the rain. One day she will limp on one leg and other day on the other; she forgets which one she uses to pretend. When I don't watch her she doesn't limp anymore. That gave away her secret."

The vet takes the file home to study which remedy would fit this peculiar behaviour of positioning herself on the edge of heights; he has never come across this behaviour. Such observations often indicate a particular remedy; it is worth then to take some extra time to find such a remedy because they usually make a significant difference for the patient.

By chance, the same evening the family watches a documentary about Musk deer in their mountains. These goats live on the edges of steep precipices; they look downwards in the same way as Nancy did in the consult room.

The remedy, Moschus, prepared from the Musk gland is known for its desire to keep in control of his life; to survive through deception.

Moschus 200K, one dose. The skin problems disappear in three weeks.

She will receive the remedy four more times over 18 months. It doesn't stop her lying on the side of heights but she doesn't fall off them anymore. Another symptom has disappeared; she used to have spasms of the nasopharynx when she was stressed.

Epilogue:

Homeopathy is a wonderful prescription technique but only really successful for the patient in the hands of practitioners who respect the patient. If one accepts its slow prescription pace there is more chance of benefiting from the smooth, rapid and lasting action of a homeopathic remedy. It is a joy to see how patients improve in their overall balance and therefore restore their life energy. Especially the benefit that old patients can have from an appropriate remedy: there are so many examples about patients ending their life in peace, shortly or a long time after they received their similimum (i.e. most appropriate homeopathic remedy).

The World Health Organisation defines health as the well being of an individual in mind, body and environment: this is exactly what homeopathy tries to obtain through classical prescription. An adequate prescription will transform a patient in such a way that the possibility of his attaining this ideal situation is greatly increased.

If you get the impression you recognise your pet in one of these cases, do not be sure that he will respond to the same remedy as that used. This is because prescriptions are often made based on small nuances that are difficult to express when cases are written up.

...a client told me...

When I went through different treatment options with a client for her ageing Labrador called Holly who suffered with long standing arthritis, of course, one of my suggestions was to search for a homeopathic remedy. After explaining how we would proceed and what she could expect we made an appointment.

This was to be a new experience for my client and the consultation went very well. At the end I explained which remedy I had selected for her dog and for what reasons. She then expressed her surprise about the things she had been able to tell me about her dog and how much we uncovered about Holly's history. The homeopathic consultation had been a very revealing experience.

She then commented that she felt she had to arrange a consultation for Poppy, the other family dog. "Otherwise it would be like sending one of your children to private school and the other to comprehensive school. That would be unfair, they would not benefit from the same chances."

...a spontaneous comment to think about...

"All truth goes through three steps: First, it is ridiculed. Secondly, it is violently opposed. Finally, it is accepted as self-evident." Arthur Schopenhauer

List of remedies.

This is the list of the remedies that appear in the cases. The page numbers between brackets refer to pages where the remedy appears in the text but not much valuable homeopathic information can be extracted.

Names and addresses of the authors of the cases

Dr. Arlette Blanchy, rue du Père de Deken 8, 1040 Brussels, Belgium

Dr. Marc Brunson, rue Vignoble 1, 4130 Esneux, Belgium

Dr. Jozeph Dabeux, Hubermont 20, 6983 Ortho, Belgium

Dr Edward De Beukelaer, Maytrees, Church Lane, Mildenhall, SN8 2LU, UK

Dr. André Doneux, 86 rue Deneumoustier, 5001 Belgrade, Belgium

Dr. André Duchamps, Rue du Corbois 79, 5580 Rochefort, Belgium

Dr. Alain Duport, La Feuillade, 17 rue Granier-de-Cassagne, 32160 Plaisance-du-Gers, France

Dr. Pierre Froment, Place du 13 Avril 1944, 07240 Vernoux-en-Vivarais, France

Dr. Loïc Guiouillier, Chemin du Vert Bois, 53370 St. Pierre-des-Nids, France

Dr Bernard Heude, rue Saint Marceau 111, 45100 Orléans, France

Dr. Didier Notre Dame, 128 rue Louis Pasteur, 76130 Mont Saint Aiguau, France

Dr. Sonja Opolka, 7 Place Montgolfier, 07270 Lamastre, France

Dr. Paul Polis, Email: paul.polis.vethomeo@wanadoo.fr (France)

Dr. Jean-Philippe Reboul, Rue de la Jacobée, 01600 Trévoux, France

Dr. Patric Rouchossé, 7 Place Montgolfier, 07270 Lamastre, France

Dr. Jean-Pierre Spillbauer, 5 rue Jules Benoit, 94360 Bry-sur-Marne, France

Dr. Luc Vandamme, 19 rue Léon Melon, 4367 Kemhexhe, Belgium

A summary of reference works.

Jacques Baur; Homéopathy, medicine de l'individu; Editions Similia, 71 rue Beaubourg, 75003 Paris, France

Jacques Baur; L'organon à travers l'histoire; Editions Similia, 71 rue Beaubourg, 75003 Paris, France

Stuart Close ; The genius of homeopathy; B. Jain Publishers,7 Wazir Pur, Ring Road, Delhi 110 052, India

Harris L. Coulter; Divided Legacy; North Atlantic Books P.O. Box 12327 Berkeley, California 94701-9998, USA

Echo's du CLH & Proceedings de Congrès; 1 rue Vignoble, 4130 Esneux, Belgium.

Samuel Hahnemann ; Organon 5th Edition; Translation and Published by Ecole Belge D'Homéopathie, Bd Louis Schmidt 91, 1040 Brussels, Belgium

Carl. G. Jung ; L'Energie psychique; Livre de poche références, Paris, France.

Moreau Jacques; Homéopathie et pragmatisme; Editions Liégeoises d'Homéopathie, 1 rue Vignoble, 4130 Esneux, Belgium.

Marchat Philippe; La médicine déchirée; Editions Privat, BP 828, 31080 Toulouse Cedex 6, France.

Prof.Dr. René Dellaert, Zijn leven en zijn werk; Soethoudt, Perenstraat 15, 2000 Antwerpen, Belgium.

Rajan Sankaran; The substance of homeopathy; Homeopathic Medical Publishers, 20 Station Road, Santacruz (W), Bombay, 400 054, India.

Jean Seignalet ; L'alimentation ou la troisième médicine; François-Xavier de Guibert, 3 rue Jean-François-Gerbillon, 75006 Paris, France.

Slauson D. O. & Cooper B. J.; Mechanisms of disease; Williams & Wilkins, 428 East Preston Street, Baltimore, Maryland 21202 USA.

Michel Zala; Consulter un homéopathe.Pourquoi? Comment? ; Edtions Liégeoises d'homéopathie, 1 rue Vignoble, 4130 Esneux, Belgium.

Printed in the United States
By Bookmasters